*Discover*
# The Secret Energized You

*Life is an experiment! What tools will you use?*

Also by Kebba Buckley

*Peaceful Joy* Meditation CD
*Receptive and Ready* Meditation CD

*Discover*

# The Secret Energized You

*Life is an experiment! What tools will you use?*

*For Virginia —*

*For the Highest and Best always —*

*Kebba Buckley Button*

Kebba Buckley, M.S., O.M.
*"The LifeTools*[sm] *Lady"*

LifeTools Press ▲ Brooks Goldmann Publishing Company, LLC

*Published by:*

LifeTools Press
Brooks Goldmann Publishing Company, LLC
7970 E. Camelback Rd. 710
Scottsdale, AZ 85251
*www.BrooksGoldmannPublishing.com*

ISBN: 978-0-9817881-0-4
ISBN: 0-9817881-0-6

# Contents

Acknowledgements ........................................... ix

Author's Note................................................... x

## Chapter 1

## Stop Fueling Your Fatigue................................ 1

Get Ready for Change ................................... 1

Push the Possibilities................................... 2

Observe Your Starting Point ....................... 4

Unshoulder Your Burdens............................ 5

# Chapter 2

# Manage Your Energy, Not Your Stress ......... 9

Understand Stress vs. Energy ....................................11
Use the Word "Stress" for Focus
Live By the UpBeat Living Energy Equation$^{sm}$

Let Stress Create Disease...Or Wellness ...................14
Court Your Master Hormone for Vitality and Youth

Get Past Old Models of Stress Management .............20

Become an Energy Manager ....................................21

Convert Negatives To Positives ...............................24

# Chapter 3

# Discover the Secret Energized You ............... 29

Create the Life Quality You Want............................29
Responsibility and Choice of State
Goals and Possibilities
The Law of Attraction
The DW2$^{sm}$ (Don't-Want-Do-Want) LifeTool
Gratitude and Go-Power
Personal Gratitude List

Use New LifeTools .....................................................37
   Put Off Procrastination
   Thank Your Body
   Love Yourself More
   Empower Yourself With Self-Talk
   Take Inspiration from Others' Qualities
   Beat Your Brain Lag

Eat For Wellbeing .....................................................45
   Eat Lovingly for Your Heart
   Maintain Your pH to Prevent Disease
   Seek Superfoods for the Super You
   Perk with Coffee
   Choose Chocolate for Health

Relate From New Views .............................................55
   Get Great Relationships with Three Top Tips
   Love in Communication Styles
   Handle Hurtful People Effectively
   Let Your Nature Nurture You
   Let Go of Advising
   Choose the B/Right Stuff
   Stump Your Stale-O-Meter$^{sm}$ with Microshift

Manage Your Moods With Energy Balancing...........70
   Center and Find Stillness
   Loosen Up
   Energize
   Release

Discharge Strong Negativity .................................73

Manage Burnout and Energy Emergencies.................75

Get Professional Bodywork/Energy Therapy ...........77

## Chapter 4

## RISE HIGHER ............................................... 85

Forgive...............................................................85

Connect...............................................................86

Change With Change ...............................................90

Carpe Diem, Not the Fish of the Day .......................92

**Resources** ........................................... 97
**Self-Quiz**............................................. 98
**Order Form**......................................... 100
**About Kebba Buckley** ................................. 101

# Acknowledgements

This book would not have been possible without the most negative and the most positive people and experiences in my life. The "negative" and "bad" people and experiences served me by spurring me to research, to learn and grow, and to develop the paradigms and LifeTools$^{sm}$ that I am sharing now. The positive people and happy experiences uplifted me, sustained me, and reminded me of the joy and full-fill-meant$^{sm}$ that is possible.

Huge thanks go to my patient and amazing book team: my cover designer, Carl Ulbrich of Jireh Communications; my publisher, Patricia L.Brooks, at Brooks Goldmann Publishing Company; my editor, Beth Phillips, the Eagle Eye Editor; my book designer, Morgan; my Web designer, Tyger Gilbert, of US Web Advertising; my reviewers, Dr. Dane Treat, Trish Turpin, Ramona Sallee, Theresa Cox, and Patricia Brooks. Endless gratitude goes to my dear friend of twenty years and my soul mate, Ron Button, whose limitless humor, love, and encouragement keep my wings aloft.

Highest praise and gratitude for the conception and completion of this book goes to the Divine, whose inspiration has filled me, my research, my skills, and these pages, from the beginning.

Kebba Buckley
"The LifeTools$^{sm}$ Lady"
2008

# Author's Note

This book is intended to provide practical LifeTools[sm] for people who want to discover their secret energized self—to reveal to themselves how much they can make of their energy, their lives, and their relationships. This book cannot substitute for, nor is it intended to substitute for, medical or counseling advice. It is hoped that each reader will consider the services of a qualified professional, if medical or counseling services are needed.

# Chapter 1

# Stop Fueling Your Fatigue

In this chapter, you will learn what actually causes fatigue. More importantly, you will learn how to stop causing your own fatigue. If situations or relationships tire you out, you can use new strategies to stop getting tired and worn. If you feel tired after eating or drinking, you can switch to taking in food and drink that is energizing for you. Through understanding and changing your choices, you can truly stop fueling your own fatigue.

## Get Ready for Change

Welcome to your personal course in discovering your true self, The Secret Energized You<sup>sm</sup>! You'll notice that I use words differently, or use new words, to get people to take a fresh look at how life works. I present ideas and methods called "LifeTools<sup>sm</sup>", throughout this book. These are not just nice ideas. They are techniques and processes for you to use to rework areas of your life where you want to discover more energy, vitality, success, joy, and transcendence. You can use LifeTools to solve negative conditions and to create positive energy. Life is an experiment! The Universe is your laboratory. What you get in life is the result of the way you have been experimenting and the tools you have been using. What tools will you use in your experiment? You must change your choices to change your results.

> **You must change your choices to change your results.**

There is a cultural idea in modern life that you can talk about a problem until you are exhausted, or your counseling budget is, and the problem will somehow go away. Actually, talking endlessly about a challenge will often magnify it. Some say, "What you resist persists". You may even overwork the problem mentally and get "paralysis by analysis". You may say, "I just want to survive this difficult time!" But I want much more for you. I want you to understand problems differently and then do things differently. I want you to thrive, not just survive. I want new results for you. I want you to fully discover The Secret Energized You.

**Aim to thrive,
not just survive.**

In live presentations, I often say, "I don't want much from you today—I just want to completely change your life!" If you read this book and use the LifeTools, you will find profound changes in your energy and the joyful dynamism of your life. Welcome to your fresh new approach to creating and living the life you want!

## Push the Possibilities

I believe that everyone can discover their secret energized self—if they want to. Using the LifeTools can take hours or as little as eleven seconds, so everyone has time to experiment with them. The paradigms shared in this book are based on timeless wisdom and the latest medical, neuro-linguistic, and psychoneuroimmunology research.

Many people are exhausted, but they don't have to be. In this quantum-paced world, do you sometimes feel overwhelmed and under the power curve? Do you feel that life is moving much faster than you are? Do you think you get sick more often, or stay sick longer, because you are "stressed out"? You are probably right. Stress affects our energy and our health in many ways. And the effects of stress can be profound and expensive. The rampant rate of autoimmune disease in this country and others is one outstanding result of the prevalence of stress. Allergies, skin irritations, fibromyalgia, fatigue, and chronic fatigue syndrome can all result from adrenal depletion and autoimmune dysfunction. Increased anger and violence in the workplace and elsewhere can also be related to unresolved stress.

In the days of cave dwellers, we needed fear to help us speed up and run away from dangers such as large predator animals. We needed anger to help us breathe deeply and feel powerful enough to run toward an enemy and fight. Warrior cultures in every age have practiced gearing up this attack chemistry so as to be brave, strong, and effective. War dances cause endocrine chemistry to flow freely, and artful war cries activate more hormone production. The aerobic exercise of running after enemies or fighting hand-to-hand burns off extra hormones and other stress chemistry.

In today's society, we are often overstimulated, responsible for too much, financially pressed, frustrated, and exhausted. Most often, we express and resolve any conflicts through words. This leaves us with a lot of unresolved stress chemistry running through our metabolisms and stored in our tissues. Thus, individuals may have stored anger chemistry from one interaction and then may appear to overreact to the next situation that "makes them angry." This has happened enough in the U.S. Postal Service that we have a modern expression, "going postal". The phrase means "losing control and becoming violent," often in response to a small stimulus. This is due to stored stress. In the U.S., health factors like high blood pressure, migraine headaches, and weight gain are at record levels. Many people have stress-caused neuromuscular pain and chiropractic issues caused by muscles in spasm. People spend billions of dollars every year on remedies for pain and exhaustion, yet most are still wondering where their energy went.

The good news is that now there are answers to these issues. If people want to handle stress more effectively, they now can literally trade it in for energy. There has never been a more complete toolkit available. Global knowledge of health care, personal self-maintenance, and issue management has now begun to merge. We now can take the best of all the international well-being toolkits and translate these many techniques into easy-to-use tools for everyone who wants them. East has met West, and meditation has met medicine. Many of these tools are included in this book as LifeTools.

So many people have been tired on a continuing basis for so long that they now think this level of fatigue may just be normal. They think it may just be something that comes with aging. Their real potential is unrevealed. It is a secret to them!

But imagine: what if your body-mind-heart-spirit system could feel energetic, renewed, and enthusiastic? What if you felt optimistic, happy, and excited about new opportunities in life? What if you were meant to live this way? As you will learn in Chapter 3, happiness, excitement, and energy lead to more production of body compounds that lead to...happiness, excitement, and energy! Imagine how energized and young you can feel and how deep your in-joy-meant[sm] can be.

As you Discover The Secret Energized You, push the possibilities. See how far the LifeTools can take you into energy, enthusiasm, and rejuvenation. You are now embarking on the most profound adventure: to Discover The Secret Energized You and redesign your life. Make the most of this adventure to make the most of your life!

## Observe Your Starting Point

So what have you created with your life experimentation up to this moment? How do you feel right now? The following is a simple way to observe what fatigue and stress you have brought in with you. Get out your pen now and start making notes as you observe yourself.

First, place a hand next to your neck, palm down. Now drop the hand to your shoulder top. You should now be at the bend that joins your neck and shoulder top. This is the first place stress lodges in the body for many people, and tightness here can control your fatigue.

How tight or loose are your shoulder muscles? Do they feel more like pudding or concrete? Privately note your stress level and assign it a score on a scale of zero ("slug" or "sandbag") to ten ("totally tight, tired and exhausted" or "poster person for espresso extreme"). Check both sides and note your score. Many of you will notice that one shoulder-top is noticeably tighter than the other. What you are measuring, at a general level, is hypermyotonia, the excessive tightness of muscle tissue due to stress. Congratulations! You have just conducted a Stress Self-Assessment! Make a note of the score you gave each shoulder and how many years old you feel. No cheating! This Stress Self-Assessment is only for you.

Gently lean your head down toward your left shoulder, then slowly raise it. Repeat to the right. Normal range-of-motion is more than halfway. Some people can stretch their head all the way to their shoulder-top. If you can't go at least halfway without straining, you have neck muscle stiffness or were possibly in an accident in the past. Make a note of how far you can lean toward each shoulder.

Now try leaning your head slowly forward, back, "northwest," "northeast," "southwest," and "southeast." Are you as flexible as you expected to be?

Does any part of your body hurt? Does it hurt regularly? Does any part of your body not work as well as it once did, other than due to injury? Does your intuition suggest that deep stress may be responsible? Or has your doctor told you directly that stress has played a role in your discomforts?

You may wish to write out a list of what you observe and consider setting goals to relax your muscles, to get back flexibility, and to investigate possible health improvements. What do you think the greatest health possibilities are for you? Would you be willing to be pleasantly surprised?

## Unshoulder Your Burdens

Here is a two-minute LifeTool that can take you straight to the Secret Energized You. Touch the top of each of your shoulders as in the previous section, and note your score on the same scale of zero to ten.

Everyone knows that stress can register in the body and make many physical areas tight, tired, or painful. You can even get sick from stress. But few know this secret: the shoulders take the biggest squeeze from stress and can be your secret weapon to unlock that stress.

We have many phrases that suggest the shoulders are a hub for stress storage in the body. We talk about "shouldering a burden" and "squaring our shoulders" to prepare for a challenge. We speak of "shouldering forward" to make progress in a competition or a thick crowd. We say, "The responsibility landed square on his shoulders."

Feel your shoulder tops again. Are they at the same index or even tighter following the discussion of what can tighten them? How old do you feel now?

We talk about "taking on the yoke of responsibility" for a long-term role or job, suggesting that "the weight of responsibility" is to be supported on the shoulders in the way that an ox or a team of oxen "shoulder the yoke" to plow forward with their work. Different kinds of thoughts lodge in different parts of our anatomy. According to Chinese medicine, the question "How am I going to solve it?" is understood to lodge in the shoulder tops, in the cross-fibers of the trapezius muscle group, and in several sets of connected neck muscles. When these muscles are tight, they squeeze on the nerves that pass through them.

Great shoulder stress then means you will have tight facial muscles. This leads, eventually, to age lines in your face. Also, ear discomfort and ringing, head pain, loss of concentration, and tooth pain can all be caused by shoulder stress. When tight shoulder-top muscles squeeze the brachial plexus nerve group, which serves the arms, this stress can cause arm fatigue and impairment of your fingers, sometimes with pain, numbness, or electric-shock sensation. General shoulder-level muscle tightness, especially over a period of time, impairs circulation to the remainder of the body and can cause great fatigue. All this will make you feel old!

So what can you do? The good news is, you can "unshoulder your burdens" to a great degree, quickly and at no cost. Unshouldering is actually easy, and you will relieve your pain, fatigue, and premature facial aging. Try this LifeTool.

1.   Run in place for two minutes. Check your shoulder-top scores, left and right. They should be down a bit.

2. Take two minutes and stretch your shoulders gently in every direction you can think of. Make it a silly game, as if you were a child getting up from one of those cramped little school desks, stretching your arms and winding them around everywhere. Feel how this movement stretches out your shoulders and how glorious that new circulation feels in your upper torso, head, and face. Check your shoulder-top scores again, left and right. They should be down one or two points.

3. For two minutes, think of anything that makes you smile and laugh, such as that goofy look your pet gives you when you run in place and stretch about strangely in your living room. Check your shoulder-top scores once more. At this point, most people's Stress Self-Assessment scores are down at least four points from their starting scores; they feel younger and healthier, and their hands are more flexible. They may feel a pleasant warmth or tingling in the feet.

Look at your initial scores and the age you said you felt six minutes ago. How young do you feel now? Turn this shoulder-loosening experiment into a twice-daily habit. Add your own variations, and soon you'll be discovering more of your secret energy and beating stress's biggest squeeze.

# Reflections

# Chapter 2

# Manage Your Energy, Not Your Stress

"The Mother of Holistic Medicine", Dr. Gladys T. McGarey (M.D., M.D.H.), has said, "Stress is probably ultimately the underlying cause of all disease."

Popular concepts of what stress is, how it works, and what can be done are leaving people exhausted. It is vital to start understanding how we can dismiss damaging outmoded ideas and use stress to our benefit. Stress, as we conventionally think of it, is destructive to health, wellness, and happiness. Instead of fighting stress or managing stress, it's time for a new paradigm. It's time to eliminate resistance and use stress as our partner in energy management. **It's time to stop managing stress and start managing our energy!**

**Figure 1, Stress Sources**, shows a range of common causes of negative stress. Are you experiencing any of these? Have you experienced these in the past?

**Figure 1. Stress Sources**

## Conflicts

Difficult People
Available Time vs. Needs and Goals
Available Resources vs. Needs and Goals
Personal Values vs. Values of an Authority Figure

## Unmet Needs

Unmet Emotional Needs
Unmet Physical Needs
Pain, Chronic Health Conditions
Limited Body Mobility
Old Emotional Agendas
Feeling Limited Or Trapped

## Unexpected External Factors

Significant Personal Loss (Human, Financial)
Significant Community Loss (Natural Disaster, 9/11 Attacks)

## Understand Stress vs. Energy

Do you want to enjoy your life more? Would you enjoy things more if you had more energy? Life today is filled with stress that most of us cannot avoid. Many people are very tired or sick from constant "stress," and they know it! Others have stress they may not recognize but which is the beginning of high blood pressure, heart disease, ulcers, cancer, diabetes, and other expensive health problems. Energy, wellness, and stress are intimately connected. If you would like to start experiencing less stress and more energy and wellness, read on!

Here is a trick question: do you think you would get more out of life if you had less stress? Most would say yes. But not all stress is the same. There is *negative stress* and there is *positive stress*. Negative stress is sometimes known as *distress*, and positive stress has been called *eustress*. It's the negative stress that steals your energy! Webster's New World Dictionary says stress is "strain; specifically force that strains or deforms; mental or physical tension; urgency, pressure, etc., causing this." Does that sound too familiar? It is the frustration, disappointment, and resistance that wear us down and help us feel bad: the too-long task list, the difficult people, the bad breaks, the information we get that is different than what we want. We call the latter "bad news."

In contrast, positive stress gives you energy, good feelings, and health. Does positive stress sound like an oxymoron? It's also known as "stimulus," "fun," "creativity," "excitement," and even "adventure." This is the set of positive forces that work, or that we operate, in our lives to shape desired outcomes in ourselves, our days, our careers, our relationships.

Imagine comparing the winning Lotto numbers with the ticket in your hand and finding that the numbers match! Your heart rate picks up and races, just as in negative-stress reactions! Your underarms and hands may sweat. Maybe you feel lightheaded or your stomach feels strange. Guess what? These are the same symptoms as when you got that audit announcement with a $5000 tax bill from IRS! Only this time, with positive stress, you have endorphins, compounds your brain releases that reduce pain and make you feel wonderful. Your sense of well-being goes up sharply. Now you have the chemistry of happiness supporting the factual good news. You have just experienced an extreme dose of positive stress.

Now here is the super news: you can deliberately add positive stress to your life to counter negative stress. Get vigorous exercise. Set up rewards for yourself for meeting goals. Join fun competitions like playing softball or board games or Nintendo. Each of these requires commitment and effort and therefore is a *stressor*, but a positive one with great rewards. Tired of fighting the monster called Stress? Take a break from the concept of monster fighting. Save that resistance effort and add positive stress to your day and your life. The negative stress will seem—and be—much less potent. You'll have more energy, feel better, and have a new investment in wellness. Start now!

## Use the Word "Stress" for Focus

When people talk about "having stress," sometimes they mean causes and sometimes they mean effects. Some people are telling you about conditions that could cause stress, and some people are describing the symptoms in their bodies. I want you to change the way you use this word "stress" now! Think of what you want to "stress," or "focus on," in your life. How do you want your life to be? Do you want to spend your life responding to annoyances? To discover The Secret Energized You, it is vital that you become an Energy Manager in your life instead of managing the stress around you.

## Live By the UpBeat Living Energy Equation<sup>sm</sup>

**Figure 2, The UpBeat Living Energy Equation**, is simple yet powerful. It illustrates how we get less overall energy by adding negative stress to our day and more energy by adding positive stress to our lives. Negative stress makes us tired, and positive stress gives us energy. What are some positives you could add to your life?

**Figure 2. The UpBeat Living Energy Equation**

$$\pm \text{ STRESS}$$

$$=$$

$$\pm \text{ ENERGY}$$

## Let Stress Create Disease...Or Wellness

**Figure 3, Effects of Increasing Negative Stress**, illustrates the many
potential negative health effects of stress if it is allowed to go
uncontrolled for too long.

One emotion that has been proven seriously damaging to our health is
anger. In biomedical studies announced in 1995, The Heartmath
Institute learned that persons who hold an angry thought of their
choosing for only five minutes have seven nervous system factors
depressed for six hours. The factors are functions of a part of the
nervous system which controls the body's immune system. Therefore,
we know *anger damages the immune system.* And how many of us,
when we have a really hot, angry thought going, limit ourselves to only
five minutes?

It is vital that we learn to see things differently and respond differently,
or learn to discharge anger. For a number of simple techniques to use,
see the section titled "Discharge Strong Negativity" in Chapter 3. You
may be surprised at how enjoyable these methods can be.

## Figure 3. Effects of Increasing Negative Stress

Mental Distress
∨
Loss of Concentration
∨
Depression
∨
Crabbiness
∨
Emotional Outbursts
∨
Physical Pains
∨
Illness and Aging
∨
Shorter Lifespan
∨
Death

Converse to the idea that the damage of stress is supposedly unstoppable, many severe health conditions have been completely reversed by reversing stress. **Figure 4, Effects of Increasing Positive Stress**, illustrates the accumulative effects of adding positives to one's lifestyle. An extreme example of this process comes from hospices in the United Kingdom. There, the emphasis is on relaxation, complete pain relief, joyful fun, and companionship. And one-fifth of UK hospice patients get completely well and go home instead of dying. Research on the body's master hormone may partially explain this phenomenon. The hormone is "dehydroepiandrosterone" (which I challenge you to say three times quickly), and is commonly known as DHEA. The following section explains the role of DHEA and the power of learning to increase your body's own production of it.

**Figure 4. Effects of Increasing Positive Stress**

# *[Pattern Repeats]*
## ⋀
# **Better Health and Vitality**
⋀
## **Greater Wellbeing**
⋀
## **Increased Energy**
⋀
**Addition of Positives**
⋀
**Better Health and Vitality**
⋀
**Greater Wellbeing**
⋀
**Increased Energy**
⋀
**Addition of Positives**

## Court Your Master Hormone for Vitality and Youth

Remember how your mama told you to go out and get some fresh air,
sunshine, and exercise? It has now been medically proven that she was
right! The master hormone, DHEA, is produced by the body when
stimulated by fresh air, sunshine, exercise, and some other simple
things. You will literally be stronger, feel better, and have greater health
if you do these things.

DHEA is produced from cholesterol, as is progesterone. However,
DHEA is used to make estrogen and testosterone. And because of
hormone production feedback loops, DHEA is a major regulator for all
other hormones, including the thyroid and pituitary functions. Ideal
DHEA levels should be at least 750 ng/dL (nanograms per deciliter of
blood) in men and at least 550 ng/dL in women.

Even if you have no formal background in life sciences, you are an
expert on one area of wellness: yours! Only you know exactly how well
you feel. Do you wake up stretching for joy and embracing how good
you feel? Or do you wake up cursing the alarm clock and wishing you
could smash it? Perhaps you have a medical diagnosis but you would
love to feel five years younger. Your DHEA levels may be the key
factor in how good you feel.

I attended a medical conference on the latest in pain-treatment research.
One of the doctors there was the famous neurosurgeon, C. Norman
Shealy, M.D., Ph.D. Dr. Shealy is known as a pioneer in the field of
pain research. He developed the TENS unit, which substitutes its
electrical impulses for your body's pain messages, greatly speeding
recovery from surgeries. Dr. Shealy is especially known for his
multimodal pain management philosophy and for founding the first
biofeedback-based pain management program in the 1970s.

What surprised and impressed me the most about Dr. Shealy's work was
his emphasis on the role of general wellness in chronic pain
management. A new paradigm of hormonal wellness has become
integral to overall well-being, following a sharp rise in research on

DHEA since the mid-1980s. Basic to hormonal balance is personal balance, which we can greatly affect for ourselves, free of charge. And for those without pain or chronic pain, the rules are the same for optimizing wellness through achieving a balance of DHEA and other, possibly more familiar, hormones.

DHEA is both an antidepressant and a cognition enhancer in patients with major depression. Dr. Shealy says that patients with every major disease have low levels of DHEA. He includes such conditions as diabetes, obesity, high blood pressure, cancer, immune deficiencies, autoimmune disorders, and coronary artery disease. Stress, whether physical, mental, chemical, or electromagnetic (e.g. computers, televisions, fluorescent lights), can deplete your DHEA rapidly. Depleted DHEA can then put you on the path to major disease conditions.

Frequenters of health food stores have been noticing DHEA supplements as one of the hot nutritional "magic bullets." But don't rush out to buy it yet! First, get your doctor to order a serum DHEA test from a lab s/he recommends. Due to uneven results from many labs, you may want to get a lab list from the American Holistic Medical Association. If your DHEA is indeed below ideal, consider some of the recent research findings and Dr. Shealy's tips for self-help. These include:

1. Learn meditation and do it thirty minutes per day. Meditators have higher serum DHEA.
2. Apply natural progesterone, such as the cream or roll-on type derived from wild yams (*dioscorea*), to the skin to raise DHEA levels. Synthetic progesterone does not provide the full spectrum of natural progesterone's biological activity, and it may have negative side effects.
3. Exercise and spend an hour a day outside or in natural light.
4. Make love more.
5. Eat a diet low in fat, very low in sugar, and with a minimum of caffeine and alcohol.
6. Don't smoke anything.
7. Keep a positive attitude.
8. Get your DHEA retested in several months.

Doesn't this list sound easy and interesting? Try these changes for even a week, and see how your vitality and happiness improve. Take two happy activities and call me in the morning.

## Get Past Old Models of Stress Management

It is vital that we see how the "regular" ways of seeing stress and stress management actually get us locked into unhelpful ways of thinking and acting. In most models of stress management, all we can do is cope with the stress or try to avoid it. Study the familiar models below, and read on to see how vital it is that we create new models for new ways of living.

> **In most models of stress management, all we can do is cope with the stress or try to avoid it. Both involve resistance, which takes energy.**

### The Stressmonster<sup>sm</sup> Model

A very popular view of stress is that it is something like a phantom or an irritating ghost that comes to visit. People say, "Oh, I really have stress today!" or "Oh, stress has really gotten to me today!" In this model, the stress is outside oneself. It is something that just happens, like weather patterns. Some people even say, "What a stressful day!" as though the stress they experience is somehow due to the day. Again, the stress is perceived as something outside themselves.

In this model, people respond like warriors fighting the phantom enemy "Sir Stress"! People say, "Oh, I'm holding up as well as I can!" But this involves resistance, which is work and which produces more stress. Therefore, people "fighting" stress get tired quickly and rarely feel they have won. You may hear these people use stronger phrases that indicate they see life as a war zone and themselves as being under siege.

### The Stress-O-Meter<sup>sm</sup> Model

In this way of thinking about stress, people see stress as heat, like a climate condition. Picture a large thermometer labeled "How hot will you get today?" As in the StressMonster Model, stress seen as is coming from outside oneself and certainly as being out of one's direct control.

In this model, people talk about "heating up" as they get stressed and "cooling off" as they unstress. They may say, "Boy, he really got hot under the collar at that meeting!" or "Yow, that's a hot topic!" or "What a heated discussion we had at that board meeting!" People may advise a stressed-out person to "cool off" or "chill out" or even "calm down" meaning "come down in your stress/heat level."

People ride up and down their personal Stress-O-Meter, the thermometer of stress, during their day. They heat up, then they cool off or chill out.     What happens when someone gets so stressed out that they hit the top of their Stress-O-Meter? They "explode" or "go over the top," just as a thermometer explodes when overheated.

How much more powerful is it to see stress as a matter of perception and focus, with each of us as the manager of our personal energy budget each day?

## Become an Energy Manager

Right now, try stretching your ideas about how to use your week. Imagine that your energy is measurable in Energy Dollars, instead of in hours and minutes. Imagine that, for each day of the week, you have a budget of 1440 Energy Dollars. That's one Energy Dollar for every minute of the day. Now imagine that it's up to you to invest your Energy Dollars wisely. You lose Energy Dollars when you invest them in people and activities that exhaust you. You multiply your Energy Dollars when you sleep really well or invest in people and activities that energize you. You have seen **Figure 1, Stress Sources**, on page 10. Review it again now, and write down a few examples of ways you became tired or energized in the last week or two. Just for fun, give your positive and negative energy investments Energy Dollar values. Do you see any patterns? Overall, are you gaining or losing energy during your week?

Stress can come from internal or external causes. We cannot fully control anything outside our own body or mind. We can, however, control our reactions (meaning "choose effective responses") to internal or external causes. We are most likely to choose effective responses and strategies if we are selecting proper breathing techniques, proper diet and fluids, best posture, best exercise regime, good sleep, and satisfying recreation.

You have seen the old models of stress management. Operating your life within these models can only lead to an exhausting life running on nervous energy. I call this The False Energy Range. In that range of energy, both fatigue and dis-ease, or "disease" will accumulate. To escape the False Energy Range, you need excellent rest, correct refueling, breathing clear air, drinking high quality water, and beginning refreshing re-creation, or "recreation." Escapees from the victimhood of exhaustion and negativity can then use LifeTools to convert stress to energy and respond more effectively to situations. This restructuring of thinking and responses then leads you into what I call The Real Energy Range. Now energy and productivity start climbing up, and the person starts to recharge, re-empower, revitalize, and actually rejuvenate.

**Figure 5, Positive Stress Sources**, illustrates some popular and effective positives you can add to your life to start to Discover The Secret Energized You. Research and try the ones that look interesting to you. Note how much energy you get from each activity. Some will probably power you up more quickly, or to a higher level, than others. Are there positives that are not in Figure 5, but which you might like to add for yourself?

## Figure 5. Positive Stress Sources

### Higher Mind/Spiritual
Prayer
Meditation
Spiritual and Religious Study
Nature Walks

### Mental
Focus On The "Now" Moment
Consultations On Effective Living Skills
Neuro-linguistic Programming (NLP)
Time-Management Principles

### Emotional
Psychotherapy
Keeping A Journal
12-Step Programs & Rational-Emotive Programs

### Physical
Diet
Supplements: Vitamins, Minerals, Herbs
Digestive Cleansing
Rest
Extra Sleep
Exercise: Dance, Sports, Yoga, Chikung
Exhaling, Breathwork
Bodywork: Massage Therapy, Energy Therapy

# Convert Negatives To Positives

So! Now you know that, without changing your life's negatives at all, you can balance them or take away their power by adding positives. Now we focus on the negatives but solely so we can discuss how to convert negative stress to energy. Do you think you don't have time for managing your stress and energy? Wrong. Two LifeTools will be covered in this section. Each will take only a few seconds. The first method applies neuro-linguistic programming, and the second uses physiology. You can begin using these immediately and continue lifelong. They do not wear out. They weigh nothing and take up no space.

The first LifeTool for converting negativity is The Problem-To-Project Switch[sm]. Neuro-linguistic programming is the science of the language of the nervous system. We can address ("talk to") the nervous system, and hence the brain stem and all physiological functions, verbally, tonally, physically, emotionally, and through facial expressions and posture. We can cause the nervous system to recall its optimum state of functioning through "keys" or "anchors," such as gestures and words. Let's take the case of language. If we use negative, heavy, emotionally loaded or jarring words, there is a negative impact on the bodymind state.

If we switch to positive, light, energetic, constructive, and connective language, we produce strong positive effects on the bodymind state. We often speak of our "problems." We say we have a "weight problem," a "money problem," a "sleeping problem," or a "personnel problem." If you chant the word "problem" to yourself for a minute, do you feel light and energetic and great? More likely, you feel weighed down and distressed. What other physiology do you feel when you focus on this common neuro-linguistic anchor, the word "problem"? If you switch to the word "challenge," what is the difference? Try chanting "challenge" to yourself for one minute. Now the fighting energy is gone, some resistance is gone, hope and optimism and reward expectation are present.

Next, try an upgrade to a higher anchor by switching to the word "project." Now you have "a health project," "an employee project," "a diplomacy project," even "a weight project." Now chant the word "project" to yourself for one minute. How do you feel? Try The Problem-To-Project Switch, and notice how much less resistance is present. Notice how much less energy each "project" takes. You have now changed the very nature of the negative stress by renaming it, and you have changed your neuro-linguistic program to handle it positively.

The second LifeTool for converting negativity is The Complete Exhale<sup>sm</sup>. In your lungs lurks an energy blockage. And you can remove it! Do you ever feel better in fresh air than in stale air? Has it been too long since you breathed fresh air, so you can't remember? Breathing well and completely, and inhaling fresh air rather than stale air, energizes the body completely when the lungs provide oxygen to the bloodstream through gas-exchange processes.

Yet few people use all of their lung capacity. Most take shallow breaths from the upper half or two-thirds of the lungs. Thus, stale air and city pollution byproducts rest undisturbed in the lower lungs. They take up space you could be using to generate physiological energy, which would increase your vitality directly.

Chinese medicine recognizes a strong relationship between joy and respiration; if you are depressed, a traditional Chinese doctor will check your "lung meridian" for lowered energy. In several cultures (India, China, Israel), the words for "breath" and "spirit" are the same. Complete breaths oxygenate and alkalize the body, making you less prone to histamine reactions. So, especially if you are depressed or allergic, augmented breathing methods are good techniques to look into. You can start by dumping the "old air load" from your lungs, thus allowing the reflexive inhale that will reload the lungs with fresh air, allowing oxygenation through the extra 50% of alveoli, or air sacs, that become available.

Now try The Complete Exhale, and do not start with a nice big inhalation! First, sit or stand up straight. Second, say the word "ha" on a tone and sustain it while exhaling deeply. Now picture your lungs

squeezing every last bit of city air pollution out of every little air sac as you exhale. Continue until you can't get a vocal sound any more.

Allow the reflexive inhale; let new air completely fill your lungs. Take a few good inhalations, picturing them filling every little air sac in your lungs. As always, observe the result. Now you have tingling skin and your shoulders have dropped! After one minute, there will be a rush up the back of your neck and head. This is the feeling of oxygen rushing to your brain! What other effects do you feel?

Repeat two times. Notice how your energy has improved? Your cheer quotient should also have risen. If you started with stress, notice how the body has relaxed? All your projects still exist, but now they drag on you less and are easier to manage. You have transformed them again by transforming your physiological state. You just moved far forward in your ongoing discovery of the Secret Energized You.

# Reflections

# Chapter 3

# Discover the Secret Energized You

I want you to live the happiest, healthiest lifestyle you can, discovering The Secret Energized You more and more. I want you to begin understanding the dynamics of health and lifestyle differently, so you can begin making different choices. Using the LifeTools in this chapter will bring your mind, body, heart, and spirit actively into the process of discovering The Secret Energized You.

**The ancestor of every action is a thought.**
**– Ralph Waldo Emerson**

## Create the Life Quality You Want

### Responsibility and Choice of State

We cannot choose all of what happens in our lives, nor can we control all of it. Some of us feel like victims of stress. When we are ready to stop being Stress Victims—when a healthy, energized, fulfilled life is more attractive than subtle victimhood—only then we begin to take responsibility for our reactions. It is then that we can start choosing how to spend our energy in our lives. We become Energy Managers rather than exhausted Stress Victims. We begin to discover the secret energized self. Will you now choose to Discover The Secret Energized You?

## Goals and Possibilities

One of the most powerful things we can do for ourselves is to be open to positive possibilities in all aspects of life. Are you willing to allow yourself to get well? Are you willing to allow yourself to achieve a promotion? Are you willing to allow yourself a massive upswing in income? Are you willing to allow yourself a happy love relationship? Have you ever noticed that there are some small or simple things you want to have in life but you don't seem to go after them? Some of them are so easy to get, yet you don't go get them. Why not? For example, many people complain about the chair they sit in the most. They say it just doesn't fit them, it's too high, it's too deep, it's too hard or unsupportive here or there. You have been in these conversations and heard the speeches. Some people can go on for years claiming they want a different desk chair, dining chair, or recliner. Do these folks act like they want to change the chair? Or do they act like people who want to talk about the chair and keep on talking about the chair? What is actually stopping the chair owner from changing the chair?

It is completely clear when we truly want something: we go after it. A morning coffee or mid-day lunch is an absolute goal, achieved daily and without fail, for many people. In larger decisions, we all know people who are sure of what they want. When their chair is not right, they try adjusting it and adding or subtracting pillows. If that doesn't meet the requirement, then they go to stores that sell chairs in their price range and start auditioning chairs. Soon, they show you their wonderful new chair, beaming at how pleased they are with the both the comfort and the problem solution. These people are open to successful changes.

The classic formula for achieving something is:

1. Set the goal.
2. Set the approximate time frame and budget.
3. Take action.
4. Stay focused until complete.
5. Enjoy your achievement.

So why do we so often fail to get to Step 3? I propose that there is a category of desire which is not a real desire. It's the category of What We Want to Want (W4). If I only want-to-want my new chair, I will not take action. I am not willing to take action. Willingness is an element for success. Inaction is not just a matter of laziness although it may appear so.

I have a short method for you to try, in three steps.

1.  Write down your goal, such as: get comfortable chair, find someone new to date, get new job, increase income by $10K per year, get rid of scars, learn to program dreams, increase stamina 50%, lose fifteen pounds without their finding me again. Note how relatively willing you are to do anything about this. Do you want it? Or do you only wish you wanted it?

2.  Write down all your reasons for achieving this goal. What payoffs will you enjoy when the goal is achieved? Again note your relative willingness to take action. It's higher now, isn't it? If not, figure out for whom this goal was really set. Was it for your parents, was it for appearances, or was it for someone else? Now, if this goal wasn't really your desire, consider setting it aside! Otherwise, proceed.

3.  Vividly picture yourself having achieved this goal, and feel exactly how good it is to have this item, condition, or achievement in your life.

Plan to repeat Steps 2 and 3 daily. Vision it! Check your relative willingness again. Wow! Are you ready now? Then it's time to stop wanting and go take action! Repeat as desired. Enjoy!

## The Law of Attraction

It is a peculiar truth that we get what we focus on. We attract what we think about. Some call this the "Law of Attraction." Unfortunately, many people are thinking about what annoys them or ticks them off or what is otherwise thoroughly undesirable. Many are thinking about how they are overweight, so they are more likely to become or stay overweight. Many are thinking they never have a good relationship or job, so they are more likely not to have a good relationship or job.

It has been shown conclusively that you are most likely to get what you want if you visualize it and affirm it. There are a number of fields that study mental optimization and offer mind-training techniques. Some of these are: neuro-linguistic programming (NLP), edu-kinesiology (Edu-K), psychoneuroimmunology (PNI), Science of Mind, and Silva Mind Control. By verbally and visually supporting their desires, people have improved their appearance, lost weight, "turned up" their immune systems to beat cancer, gotten stress symptoms under control, quit addictions and lost the cravings, improved their sex lives, and shifted their achievements and relationships to get the results they wanted.

Try the exercise below for three days. However, before you start the exercise, here are some tips to make it more effective:

1.  Record your observations and results, even if they don't "fit" on the chart.

2.  Decide if you would like to do this for another three days.

3.  If you are still investing significant time or energy in "Don't wants", repeat steps 1–3 until you automatically catch and reverse the "Don't-wants" into "Do-wants".

4.  If you have to take extra time to consider the "Do-want" that goes with a "Don't-want," just record the "Don't-want" and take all the time you need within the three days. It is important to make some selection of a "Do-want" for each "Don't-want," even if you change or upgrade it later! This is your exercise, with your best results!

## The DW2$^{sm}$ (Don't-Want-Do-Want) LifeTool

Thoughts are things. Notice whenever you are thinking of something you do or don't like or want. Record these preferences in the columns below. When you find a "Don't-like" or a "Don't-want," flip it and say what the opposite is. Say what you do want. How much attention are you giving to the negative versus the positive? Since negative attracts negative, writing the positive opposite is vital!

For a concentrated experience, sit for fifteen minutes, simply thinking about the kind of life you want. Record everything that comes to you about yourself, people, characteristics, conditions, and places. When you finish this exercise, you will have a clearer picture of the overall life you want.

Use all the paper you want. Repeat the exercise until you are bored with it. Now, in the circuitry of consciousness, you have activated the life you truly want. Repeat the exercise every few months and notice changes.

I DO LIKE  +                                   I DON'T LIKE +
I DO WANT                                      I DON'T WANT

_____              _____

## Gratitude and Go-Power

By now, you are catching this theme: **emphasize the positive to fade the negative**. Of course, there are many ways to deal with negatives. You probably also remember that **optimum stress management is really personal energy management**. And what we most need is energy. So here, we are including as "negatives" anything that takes your energy, together with anything that you allow to take your energy. Notice our wording: yes, it suggests that we sometimes allow negative "energy sinks" to sap us.

These energy sinks can be the black holes of personal energy management! Some of them are: negative people, negative moods, the "bad breaks" we get, negative events (*i.e.,* outcomes conflicting with our desires), "bad" weather, and most of all, our own negative thoughts.

What? Our own thoughts are draining our energy? Absolutely! Over a long period of time, your negative thoughts and feelings can make you sick and create major diseases.

When was the last time you felt great while experiencing jealousy? How about fear? How about insecurity causing jealousy (you caught it—it's the same thing)? Does anger feel good? Is depression wonderfully uplifting and energizing? Do you feel nice and relaxed in a state of embittered resentment? Obviously, fun, joy, and excitement are better energizers.

Not only do your negative thoughts drain you, but they drain others and erode your relationships. Are there people you now avoid because of their negativity? Good! Don't let them drain you! Ask yourself, "Do I sometimes notice people steering clear of me?" It would be a tough thing to admit, but many of us, at times, have driven others off with our clinging to negative thoughts, feelings, and communications. Some even engage in "joy-bashing," deliberately trying to swiftly bring down someone who is feeling good and making positive statements.

Here's one simple antidote to your negative thoughts: practice gratitude. Many negative thoughts boil down to (petulantly?) resenting what we don't have or fearing we will lose what we do have, financially, emotionally, or physically. But assessing the full delight of that which we do have can invoke a marvelous state.

Anyone who has gone bankrupt and rebuilt their finances knows the delicious wonder of being able to pay the electric bill in full and on time. In this light, we can then be grateful for our bills, even our taxes! Your car may not be a late model Jaguar, but you can be grateful for its wonderful dependability and that it's completely paid for. A city transit system may be inconvenient generally and virtually unavailable on Sundays. Having a car, you can at least drive your happy heap where you want to go—on Sunday or any other day. Choose gratitude for your geographic freedom.

So, you don't have the Love of Your Life? You do have the love of wonderful friends, Mom, your dog/cat/fish, and God. Some say God loves you whether you want God to or not; that's tenacity! Are people just not catering to you? Volunteer for a charity a few hours a month and feel that incredible paradox, the getting that comes from giving. Is the world just not giving you the recognition/lifestyle/job/sex/whatever that you want? So be grateful for the freedom to make of your life what you want it to be! Get proactive and create what you want.

Do you feel unappreciated and unthanked for your efforts at home, on the job, in your clubs? Actually, most people have no idea of your efforts, not even your supervisor. Start thanking individuals and organizations for things they do that make a positive difference to your life. Here's another apparent paradox: thanking generates thanking and the feeling of oneself being more appreciated. So keep those thank-you cards and calls flowing!

> **Joy in looking and comprehending is nature's most beautiful gift.**
> **—Albert Einstein**

Do you not have much money these days? You don't even need a coupon for these freebies: blue sky and clouds, the moon and stars, a nighttime walk, the smell of flowers or pine trees, the first morning stretch, hair, the sound of a breeze rustling leaves, a baby's smile, a friend's hug, the glistening of a lake, the quiet of new snow, the phone ringing with a friend on the other end. To start feeling great again, think of all you do have. Start keeping a list or gratitude journal. You'll notice that, the more items you list that you're grateful for, the more you will think of as you write. Soon you'll know that you're going to need a long piece of paper or a journal book. Following is a LifeTools format, the Personal Gratitude List, with examples to get you started with this process.

Personal Gratitude List

Dear God, Dear Source, Dear Universe, Dear Self, [pick one]

I am very grateful for all these things: [add your choices]

      freedom
      love
      my favorite church
      blue sky and clouds
      the moon and stars
      a nighttime walk
      the smell of flowers or pine trees
      the first morning stretch
      hair
      the sound of a breeze rustling leaves
      a baby's smile
      a friend's hug
      the glistening of a lake
      the quiet of new snow
      the phone ringing with a friend on the other end
      seeing a fine movie
      coffee with a friend
      a drive in the country
      fresh flowers

# Use New LifeTools

The more a person feels whole and complete, the more whole and complete her/his relationships can be. The more complete a person is inside, the more complete s/he is in relationships with "the outside". Use the next few sections to increase your sense of wholeness. Then watch your relationships change, becoming easier and more pleasant.

## Put Off Procrastination

Think for one complete minute about what you want in your life. What professional, personal, and fun conditions do you wish were true for you? I'll wait. And now think, for one complete minute: what have you been doing about it? I'll wait.

Okay, time's up. If you noticed a gulf between what you say you want, and what you go after, have you considered you may be a procrastination pro? Do you often put off until later a useful or necessary task you could very well do today? Would you succeed better in your job or relationships if you completed tasks in a more timely way? Do you lose opportunities because you just don't apply yourself or otherwise step up? "Procrastination" generally means "deferring" or "delaying," perhaps until an opportunity is lost. Its origin goes back to at least the 1500s, with the root *crastinare* relating to a Latin word for "tomorrow." Clearly, this is not a new, modern problem. So why would anyone put off doing something that will give them the payoff they say they want?

The late Arizona State University professor Mervin Britton believed that people hold themselves back because of six types of fears. In his book, *Willingness, The Driving Force of Accomplishment*, he identified:

1. Fear of failure
2. Fear of others' judgment
3. Fear of not being right
4. Fear of not looking good
5. Fear of unworthiness
6. Fear of success itself

A person who does not have these fears, or who has conquered them, will be more willing to seek success and satisfaction. The less-fearful person will be less likely to procrastinate.

Many authors link extreme self-expectations with depression and self-defeat. Perfectionism is seen by many researchers as an expression of fear—of failure, of others' judgment, of not looking good…a familiar list. People with fears may seek to make themselves or their work "perfect" before putting it forth. Never reaching "perfection," they never complete, submit, apply, or ask that person out. There is even a book targeting this mechanism in the gifted: *Perfectionism and Gifted Children*, by Rosemary Callard-Szulgit.

But what if you are not in fear? What if everything you need to do is well within your range, but you are just not getting it all done? Perhaps you are not a procrastinator, and it's time to look at your productivity and your commitments. Can you be more efficient, take fewer birthday lunches, watch fewer DVDs for fun? Do you simply need to promise less? Or do you need to reprioritize some of your professional activities? Can you take a year off from one of those nonprofit boards? Can you go to just half the meetings of one or two professional organizations? Can you cut your mentoring practice in half? Or what about eliminating all meetings and volunteering for six weeks while you catch up on the work you get paid for?

**What are you willing to do for the life you say you want?**

Are you a procrastinator? Perhaps. Look back at your answers from the exercise in paragraph one. Now maybe you are *willing* to step up differently to get different results. Ask not what your life can do for you; ask what you are willing to do for your life.

Thank Your Body

Your body is incredibly complex and miraculous. Blessedly, we don't have to give it instructions to breathe or to pump blood or to conduct many other processes. Try to imagine living a normal day if you even had to tell your lungs when to inhale and exhale. Now picture a trillion cells, each with many processes going on inside them. The brain, via the nervous system, regulates all that. Now think about all the times you fell down and went boom before age five. Think of how hard you hit the ground and all the body parts you tore or broke. It is amazing so many of us lived beyond age five, let alone are still able to wave our arms and legs, see, walk, talk, and think fairly well. The body has amazing recuperative powers.

Now think about some of the stressors you've asked your body to handle as an adult: all-nighters, partying with alcohol and maybe drugs, simple overeating to the point of pain. Perhaps you have been hiking the Grand Canyon without conditioning your dear, loyal body first. Perhaps you smoke, whatever materials. Certainly you have professional stresses, conflicts, overloads, and difficult people to deal with.

Yet your body keeps carrying you around. If you talk nicely to it, it will function at a higher level. If you talk to it in a mean way, it will function at a lower level. This is a part of neuro-linguistic programming (NLP), or psychoneuroimmunology (PNI): what you say, your body believes, because your messages are carried by the nervous system to all parts of the body. Your word actually becomes your bond with the body.

So how do you talk to your body? Do you call it ugly, fat, or slow? What comments do you make to yourself when you first look in the mirror in the morning? Now change your self-talk and thank the body for everything good you can think of. Thank it for carrying you around faithfully, for accepting pizza and diet soda as "dinner" night after night. Thank it for sleeping efficiently, for reproduction, and for pleasure. Thank it for growing such nice hair. Tell your body it has a super immune system and how grateful you are for its vigor, and you will be amazed at how great you feel. Thank your body every morning and many other times.

Love Yourself More

In a related phenomenon to gratitude for the body, self-love is a very powerful weapon in your war on stress and your quest for energy. Many of us not only do not feel grateful for life, and for being alive, but we actually hate ourselves. If you doubt it, listen to what people say about and to themselves. We have some very hateful self-talk. For example, some have been taught to stand in front of a mirror, naked, and tell themselves how ugly they are, as a technique to assist in weight-loss programs. Even without such training, many have been told they are ugly, stupid, clumsy or incompetent, by people in frustrated moods. Negative self-talk is not just destructive "psychology." This kind of language has profound effects on your body. Change your self-talk to the way you wish loved ones would talk with you. Your brain and your nervous system are listening, and your language will lodge in your body.

Another answer is in treating yourself like you wish dear ones would treat you: gently, kindly, with sweet and affirming words, with rewards, and with hot baths by candlelight. Is there a fine sherry you wish someone would give you a bottle of? Then buy one for yourself. Many people buy themselves a fine gift for Valentine's Day. Why wait? Why not buy it today? Do you need time to yourself? Then book it. Commit to yourself to have some solo time, work out the details, and then keep that commitment.

If you would like a quick yet powerful NLP shortcut, try this LifeTool. On waking and on lying down to sleep, say "I love myself unconditionally" twenty-five times. Do it constantly while going for a walk or in another automatic activity. Notice the difference. Your attitude and your body will soften up. You have just moved closer to gentle and fabulous health.

Empower Yourself With Self-Talk

Are you ready for an intermediate exercise? Then pick six of the following expressions, developed by the author, to build your own morning/evening self-speech. If a phrase in the list below is irrelevant to you, ignore it. When you have compiled your six expressions, make two copies, one for your wallet and one for your bedside table. Read your expressions to yourself morning and evening. Try this for two weeks. Notice everything starting to go your way. Enjoy it!

*I love myself unconditionally. I'm a precious Child of God (Expression of the Divine).*

*I'm a powerful woman who walks in Grace and beauty (man who walks in wisdom and authority).*

*I'm in perfect, young, beautiful, radiant health. I love my slim, strong, energetic body. My body easily metabolizes whatever I eat or drink; it takes the best and lets go of the rest.*

*I have excellent discernment (not judgment) and easily make the wisest decisions for my life. I always know how to best allocate my time and energy.*

*My mind is always clear. I focus easily and complete tasks very efficiently.*

*Any appearance of clutter in my life and space is now substantially reduced. I love how clearing clutter clears my mind and clearing my mind clears clutter.*

*In every moment, I do my best, as I have always done my best in every moment of life. I know deeply that others are doing their best also. I feel, at least, compassion for all people and situations. All Life is connected, and I am connected to All Life.*

*I'm a complete success, financially and in all ways. I am a superb steward of my finances and of all my resources.*

*I have a core, deep within me, of profound and limitless personal peace. I know I am on my perfect life path.*

*I have and build strong, joyous relationships with my family and everyone. I feel safe and secure. I feel worthy, well-liked, and loved. My heart is full and happy. I count! I am needed.*

*The perfect friends, colleagues, and opportunities are always flowing easily into my life.*

*I love my life!*

## Take Inspiration from Others' Qualities

Where do you get your inspiration? Think about the moments when you say to yourself, "Now that is something I want to do/be/have in my life!" Many people inspire us with the qualities they embody. When we see what they have created and achieved, and when we see how they live, we are uplifted or excited, or we may even see the solutions to challenges in our own lives.

Many school children in the United States are taught the quality of honesty through a story of George Washington's life. As a child, he is said to have chopped down a cherry tree and then proclaimed, "I cannot tell a lie; I chopped it down." He went on to play a leading role in the founding of our country. His life inspires me most because he was a professional farmer who preferred not to lead. He reluctantly took up the mantle of loyal duty to a new country, serving in revolution and in new peace, never forgetting his passion to go back to Virginia and manage his farmlands.

George Vanderbilt and Frederick Law Olmstead were two stars of visionary green living design in the late 1800s. George was a nerd of his time, with health challenges that prevented him from having a regular career in his family's skyrocketing shipping business. He studied and traveled the world, and eventually he developed a vision of a self-sustaining estate as a home for his family. Frederick Law Olmstead, the designer of New York City's Central Park, believed natural-looking landscape makes the finest design. Olmstead joined Vanderbilt in the venture of creating a 125,000-acre kingdom now known as "Biltmore" in Asheville, NC. The "countryside" surrounding the 125-room, 4-acre mansion is entirely designed and landscaped for beauty, inspiration, and sustained biosystems. The house, dairy, winery, and extensive grounds remain privately owned by the Vanderbilt descendants. The kingdom and the vision are consistent with today's values of green communities.

I have long admired people who were serious achievers in their professions, yet consistently maintained a pleasant, light-hearted manner. My favorite role model for light cheerfulness blew into the world of television in the 1960s. Portrayed by actress Diana Rigg, British crime investigator Emma Peel always maintained a light, cheerful, punny, brief manner, while using judo to flip the bad guys over her petite shoulders and save the day together with her professional partner, nearly equally cheerful crimebuster John Steed. They would have a little drink and shrug off the day with a quick, light quip, then drive off into the British countryside. Reruns of that show, *The Avengers*, still air on BBC America, and DVDs of their adventures are enjoying brisk sales 40 years after production ceased. Perhaps others found the upbeat competence inspiring.

How about the quality of organization? Did you ever think you would live better if you were more organized? Then consider perhaps the reigning contemporary model for organized living, Marla Cilley, more familiarly known as "The FlyLady." She began with a nightly sink-cleaning routine and has evolved into a lifestyle guru, urging women and others to improve their home- and life management using streamlining methods. If you also admire the quality of organization, many recommendations of The FlyLady are available at no cost, on her website, *www.flylady.net*.

As you read about these people who embody different qualities, did you feel curious, uplifted, oddly happy, or excited to learn more about them? What other qualities and inspiring people come to mind for you? Why not make notes, find your inspiration, and start incorporating those qualities more into your own life? Why not enjoy your best life now?

## Beat Your Brain Lag

Everyone has a sense that their mind affects their well-being. This is never more clear than when the mind isn't—clear, that is. People sometimes notice that their memories seem to work less well than in the past. Sometimes numbers seem harder to manipulate, words are harder to recall, or a person picks up the wrong object. Sometimes we arrive in a room and wonder why we went in there. Sometimes we can't remember the name of someone we know well. Most of the time, these slips of mental clarity are transient and unimportant. Sometimes, these moments build into annoyances. If loved ones are expressing concern, this memory loss may even signal the beginning of a clinical condition.

The first remedies for slight memory/clarity impairment are inexpensive, simple, and quick to try. Try these this week:

1.  Get enough sleep. Do you? Different people need different amounts of sleep.

2.  Drink more water. The brain needs to be well hydrated for proper electrical conductivity and for the left and right hemispheres to communicate well with each other.

3.  Get some daily exercise, such as walking for 20 minutes. The resulting boost to the circulatory system may be all you need.

4.  Eat lots of fresh fruits and vegetables. The enzymes and other nutritional factors may fill in gaps in your brain's neurochemistry.

5.  Drink less alcohol. Any alcohol consumption reduces memory function, according to Dr. Stephen Flitman, Medical Director of 21st Century Neurology in Phoenix, AZ. In the long term, alcohol abuse leads to brain dehydration and shrinkage. You can always try a no-alcohol regime for two weeks and just see if your mind is clearer.

If the first five steps don't clear your mind enough, express your concerns to your doctor, who may recommend lab tests to see what may be out of balance. You may have an allergy, Vitamin B or mineral deficiency, or clinical depression. A simple thyroid imbalance or infection factors can imitate or cause the beginning of a dementia condition. Today, more is known than ever before about the diagnosis and treatment of brain conditions. In the last decade, there have been remarkable advances in neuroscience, and the brain's functions and dysfunctions are known in astonishing detail.

Whatever the extent and cause of your brain lag, if it's annoying, do research it right now. Invest in your future mind. You may find complete relief and a whole new level of The Secret Energized You. Enjoy your new clarity!

# Eat For Wellbeing

### Eat Lovingly for Your Heart

My friend Ray worked in a hospital. In fact, he worked in a famous heart-transplant unit. He had worked, typically, sixty to eighty hours a week since going to work for the heart surgeon fifteen years before. Ray was a wiry, brilliant, energetic, and good-humored man, who obviously had a passion for his work. No one thought of him as anything but incredibly healthy.

One day, Ray suddenly collapsed. His chest pain was incredible, and he couldn't catch a breath well enough to shout for help. Staff saw him sinking to the floor, writhing and gesturing, but they thought he was kidding. A couple of them laughed and said, "Good one, Ray!" How could this vigorous man be having a cardiac event? Fortunately, Ray's colleagues overcame their shock and went to work on him.

A devout workaholic and a bon vivant in his few off hours, Ray had managed to accumulate coronary blockages. Since that day, Ray has cut back his work hours, switched to a low-fat diet, started systematic exercise, and even learned some relaxation techniques. His health is excellent.

Unlike some body parts, the heart is not optional equipment. Think about it. Many of you have may have had your tonsils, adenoids, appendixes, and/or gallbladders removed for troublemaking. Noses have been trimmed and chins filled out. Tubes have been clipped and arteries cleared, stented, or bypassed. There is much anatomy and physiology you can do without or supplement, but the human system still needs a functioning heart to pump the blood, or breath stops and so does life.

So, what can you do to avoid sudden trauma like Ray had? Focus on saving time, trouble, and money by preventive maintenance of your health. Try the metaphor of "banking health" as you explore the best diet, exercise, relaxation techniques, and occasional health tests for your lifestyle. A great resource website is *www.americanheart.org*, the site of the American Heart Association (AHA). You can register and track your progress, if scoring yourself is fun for you, at the AHA website.

The AHA recommends diet changes that trend away from saturated fats and fast foods to lean meats and fish, green veggies, dark green leafy salad, and colorful fruit. Many recipes and even recipe books are available to help keep you from Righteous-Food Boredom. Many fast-food companies now have low-fat sandwiches and salads with low-fat dressings. Make this change alone, and you'll find your energy increasing and your skin looking younger. Could good health be, um, something that actually feels good?

Other changes to consider include lessening negative stress and beginning pleasant exercise. If you currently smoke anything or drink quarts of alcohol each week, this is not lessening your negative stress. It's actually poisoning you. It's also putting a huge load on your blood biochemistry and your heart. A little red wine contains compounds that can actually help the heart, as do red grapes and cocoa powder. Now, do not go out and tell people I suggested you eat chocolate candy, which can contain a lot of saturated fat. If you love chocolate, read the section later in this chapter on the health benefits chocolate can provide.

Finally, do consider actually seeing your medical doctor for a checkup. S/he has put in many thousands of hours to qualify for treating and advising patients and to maintain his/her expertise. At least get your blood pressure checked. You may prevent time-consuming, crippling, and expensive health events. And who knows? The worst that could happen is that you'll discover that you and your heart are champions of health. Be a champion: love your heart into great health.

## Maintain Your pH to Prevent Disease

Many people would make one or two easy changes in their daily habits if they could feel much better as a result. Are you one of them? Here are some points to ponder regarding a condition affecting many people and causing silently deteriorating health, yet which you can easily and inexpensively control. It's called acidosis, meaning excess acid in the body's fluids. Relative acidity is measured on the pH, or potential hydrogen, scale that indicates hydrogen ion concentration. The pH scale goes from 1 (extremely acidic) to 14 (extremely basic, or alkaline). The body operates best when its pH is between 7.35 and 7.45, ideally at 7.4. Yet diet and stress tend to acidify the body's fluids. Accumulation of biochemical waste in the body can also lower pH.

While the condition is simple, the symptoms are many. A person with acidosis may experience frequent fatigue, allergies, bronchitis, colds and flu, foot fungus, acne, boils, eczema, age spots, arthritis, diarrhea and/or constipation. Effects less easy for the individual to see are serious internal processes, such as the inflammation of veins, arteries, and the muscle tissue of the heart. This creates cardiac system issues that result in elevated blood pressure, which in turn increases the deterioration.

Acidosis also leads to premature aging via accelerating free-radical damage to cells. Cells are actually poisoned by inefficiently eliminated cellular waste. An acidic pH prevents the proper storage and release of cellular energy, meaning that the body cannot respond fully to stress or infection. Red blood cells clump together, which limits their oxygen-carrying capacity and leads to fatigue and weakness. Cancer cells thrive in lower-oxygen environments such as acidosis can create. Other mechanisms caused by acidosis may lead to pancreatic dysfunction, diabetes, weight gain, and osteoporosis.

The body has natural mechanisms for monitoring and controlling its acid-base balance. When plasma is too acidic, the respiratory system speeds breathing, and the kidneys can produce substances that turn the pH around. The body also uses intracellular absorption of hydrogen atoms by molecules of protein, phosphate, and carbonate in bone, thus raising the pH to less acidity.

So what can you do to help yourself beat acidosis? First, get litmus paper from your pharmacy and test your saliva. The litmus paper will turn color to indicate the acidity of your saliva. If your saliva's pH is too low/acidic, re-assess your current stress, exercise (or lack thereof), and diet. Consider these dietary changes:

1.  Stop drinking any sodas or sugared drinks, or any artificially sweetened products. Switch to juices or filtered water.
2.  Stop eating sugared desserts and foods made mainly with white flour and yeast, such as pizza and bagels.
3.  Eat dark-green leafy salads, other green vegetables (broccoli, cabbage, celery, parsley), and root vegetables (carrots, yams, daikon radish).
4.  Eat fruits, especially fresh fruits, such as apples, apricots, bananas, cantaloupe, dates, figs, grapefruit, peaches, and grapes. For dried fruit, try raisins.
5.  Eat rice and buckwheat, almonds, dairy products, and eggs.

Try changing your diet for a week, and add rhythmic breathing exercises. Check your pH again. Notice if these changes make you more relaxed, clear-minded, and vital. If so, you are making a major investment in your long-term health. Why not feel your best, starting now?


## Seek Superfoods for the Super You

Food has changed in recent decades, and we must now choose what to eat more by informed choice than by craving. With large-scale farming and food production, and with the prevalence of processed food in microwaveable dinners, the nutrition in typical meals has plummeted. Food is delicious, you eat more, and you get... a drop in energy! You gain weight, you feel tired, you crave carbs, and you are baffled. Sometimes you wonder, "Is this dragging feeling just from getting older?" Most people are saying, "I just wish I had more energy!"

Each person has about 70 trillion cells in the body, and all those cells want more energy. It feels like it, too, doesn't it? And remember, your body has only what you put in your mouth as material to make all your new cells.

So what can you add to your diet to get the energy you want? How about the new classes of *superfoods* or *functional foods*? These are the ones you eat not because you are hungry, but because you want to enhance sports performance, strengthen metabolic functions, or simply have more energy. The natural superfoods are single-ingredient foods, with astronomical nutritional properties, like broccoli, blueberries, or the mangosteen fruit.

More powerful are the new combined or *engineered superfoods*. In the last decade, the power of natural *antioxidant* fruits has been widely marketed. *Antioxidant* compounds fight *free radicals* and the aging they cause. **Figure 6, Superfood Terms**, gives more details of what these expressions mean.

# Figure 6. Superfood Terms

*Antioxidants:* nutritional substances that fight the oxidative deterioration of tissue. They have an "anti-aging" effect.

*Free radicals:* molecules with an odd, unpaired electron, ultimately causing cell damage; a key cause of aging. These are very unstable and react quickly, attacking the nearest stable molecule to "steal" its electron. This creates a new free radical and starts a chain reaction that disrupts a living cell. Free radicals can be created by the body to assist immune functions. However, they are often created by environmental factors such as pollution, radiation, cigarette smoke, and herbicides.

*Functional foods:* foods or dietary components that may provide a health benefit beyond basic nutrition. Foods eaten to solve a health issue. *Superfoods.*

*Oxidation:* in the body, a type of tissue-damaging process. *Free radicals* cause it, and *antioxidants* work against it.

*Phytonutrients:* nutrient compounds that come from edible plants, especially fruits.

*Superfoods:* foods with special health-promoting properties. *Functional foods.*

*Stem cells:* special cells made by the body, which can develop into any of many types of cells. They serve as a repair system for the body. There are two types, *embryonic* and *adult stem cells.* There is great debate over the use of stem cells from embryos for research.

Thanks to the globalization of communications and trade, nutrition scientists have found fruits in India, Brazil, and other countries, that have extreme antioxidant properties. Combinations of such fruits are being developed as pleasant beverages for maximum health benefits. Biologists have learned to create delivery systems in vitamin-mineral combinations, to disperse different nutrients, once swallowed, to the parts of the body where they will be the most powerfully utilized. Chemists are engineering super-waters. Biologists have found lake plants that can provide powerful nutritional and health benefits. Combined and engineered superfoods have now become widely available.

Wow! As lifestyle speeds are zooming, the world of energy nutrition and superfoods is also racing joyfully into the future. In your real life, amid the vast constellation of supplemental nutrition products, which should you run to try?

First, of course, check with your doctor, to see if your body is especially low in potassium, iron, blood glucose, thyroid function, or another health component. Then, try one superfood at a time until you find the effects it can have for you. Different people have different metabolisms, so each of us needs to experiment for ourselves. Can you feed superfoods to your child? Yes, usually you can, according to the child's body weight. Just check with the source company or your pediatrician first, since a child's metabolism has different needs than that of an adult.

Here are four of the newest, most promising superfood products:

1. **MonaVie™.** Available as a liquid or a gel, it's formulated for a one- to two-ounce daily portion. MonaVie is made primarily from the juice of the Brazilian Açai berry, the top antioxidant berry known to science (*http://www.berrydoctor.com/broadcast/2008/ORAC2008.htm*), plus eighteen other nutrition-packed fruits. Unlike many antioxidant fruit drinks, this one is delicious. Many who drink it say they feel more energy, nap less, feel more clear minded and vital within a day or two, and have softer, smoother skin. A medical study of MonaVie™ (*http://www.aibmr.com/monavie.pdf*) indicates that it inhibits the oxidation of cholesterol, slowing the process by which cholesterol

becomes more damaging. More studies are to come. For more information, or to find the product, go to *www.monavie.com*.

2. **Vitalizer.** Now you can quit hunting through health-food stores for a collection of nutrition products to shake out of jars every morning. In one convenient "Vita-strip®," six caplets and capsules provide a combination of vitamins, minerals, probiotics, Omega-3 fatty acids, and bioflavonoids. Designed by doctors for the Shaklee® Corporation, this one is designed for timed release of each component. Take it with breakfast. Those who are taking it report feeling more energy, strength, stamina, and mental clarity the first day, plus general strengthening over a period of weeks, increased wellness, and even reduced allergies.

   A recently published landmark study (*http://www.shaklee.com/NewsRelease07_102907.shtml*) shows that users of this Shaklee multiple supplement had markedly better health than other groups studied. The long-term study found the Shaklee supplement users to have higher blood levels of key nutrients, more optimal levels of key health biomarkers, and lower prevalence of diabetes and elevated blood pressure. More studies are planned. For more information, or to get Vitalizer, go to *http://www.shaklee.net/energizedyou/prodVitalizer*.

3. **i-H₂O, or i-water.** This is the most innovative liquid product I have ever encountered. Simply explained, i-H$_2$O is engineered water for use as a skin spray or for drinking. In a proprietary process, the water molecules have been organized to behave differently toward each other than they do in normal water. This results in greater absorption, calming, and healing of skin when the water is used as a spray, and energizing and tending to heal other modern ailments when used as a drink. There are no added ingredients. Some say they can feel a distinct energizing effect from just holding the bottle. The manufacturer believes that the product assists the body in fighting the effects of electromagnetic frequency (EMF) pollution. While there are not yet medical studies, it is exciting to think of the potential of this product at the cellular level, and over the long-term, for health and vitality. Find out more or get some to try at *www.myBIOPRO.com/helenspierce*.

4. **Stem Enhance®.** This product arrives as capsules to swallow with or without meals, once or twice a day. This is a patented blend of two botanical components extracted from a type of freshwater plant, *Aphanizomenon flos-aquae* (AFA). This is the product that can possibly end the issue of legalizing the commerce of embryonic stem cells. It stimulates the release of a person's own stem cells from the bone marrow into the bloodstream, potentially causing healing of serious conditions over a period of time. Those who take it speak glowingly of losing their fatigue and even their chronic fatigue. Since stem cells go to whatever body system needs help, adherents find improvement in a wide variety of conditions. When the medical studies are done, this one should win a Nobel Prize in Medicine for revolutionizing personal vitality enhancement and ending the moral debate over embryonic stem cells. To learn more about this astonishing product or to access it, go to *http://www.stemtechbiz.com/about_sub_orig.aspx.*

## Perk with Coffee

Coffee lovers worldwide know the distinctive aroma, taste, and general effects of a steaming—or iced—cup of this ancient beverage. Served black, thick with spices, or dressed up with milk, cream, foam, soymilk, sugar, and possibly flavored syrups, coffee is the beverage of choice for millions. Entrepreneur upstart Starbucks, now the industry leader in the U.S., even sponsors coffee shops on the Mercy Ships, floating surgical hospitals serving the African coastal countries with free medical services.

So, aside from taste, why is coffee so popular? Any coffee drinker will tell you they get a short-term boost from drinking java. They would all agree with the medical studies that have proven that coffee produces an increase in energy and mental clarity, including memory, for an hour or more after it is consumed. Many assume that boost is from the caffeine in the cup. In conversation, people often refer to coffee and caffeine as though caffeine is the only substance in coffee. These folks believe coffee is simply a stimulant and a metabolic cheat. The truth is much more beneficial and enjoyable.

According to the *American Journal of Clinical Nutrition* (*AJCN*), the antioxidants in coffee may reduce inflammation and thereby reduce the risk of potential disorders related to it. Cardiovascular disease is one of these. Phenols, volatile aroma compounds, and oxazoles in coffee contribute to its high antioxidant content. Researchers were surprised to discover that coffee is the single major contributor of antioxidants to the diet of both U.S. residents and Norwegians. A typical serving of coffee contains more antioxidants than typical servings of grape juice, blueberries, raspberries, and oranges, according to another study in the *AJCN*.

The *Journal of the American Medical Association* (*JAMA*) published a broad review of studies of coffee use. Coffee is now known to be associated with a lower risk of Type 2 diabetes, as well as lower risk of heart disease, liver cancer, and cirrhosis of the liver. Drinking decaffeinated coffee produced the same results as drinking coffee with its inherent caffeine, up to five cups per day. However, researchers are not suggesting that people raise their coffee intake in order to prevent disease. Of course, everyone needs to coordinate self-medication with their doctor or other medical professional.

So do you love coffee? Do you feel good, feel alert, and function well with a cup or three per day? Then why not relax in a favorite chair, drink your favorite blend, and let the research roll in?


## Choose Chocolate for Health

Here is good news for chocolate lovers: in ways, chocolate is good for you! A surprising number of studies in the last few years have examined the health benefits of chocolate. Here's what we know right now.

Chocolate, as we usually eat it, is a confection made of cocoa, cocoa butter, sugar, lecithin as an emulsifier, and flavorings. Sometimes it contains milk, as in "milk chocolate." Cocoa contains hundreds of nutritional components including the vital minerals copper, calcium, iron, potassium, and magnesium. Cocoa also contains serotonin and phenylethyalanine, two natural brain compounds that create a sense of well-being. A compound called *theobromine*, a cousin to caffeine, is another component that gives people a sense of boost after eating chocolate. Further, cocoa contains powerful antioxidants, principally *flavonol,* a polyphenolic compound that optimizes cell metabolism. *Polyphenols* are the same great antioxidants proven beneficial for cardiac function as well as others, in studies of the effects of drinking red wine and green tea. *Flavonoid compounds* reduce the stickiness of platelets, which slows blood clotting and reduces the danger of coronary artery blockages. Chocolate also contains *stearic acid,* a type of fat that doesn't raise cholesterol levels.

According to the *American Journal of Clinical Nutrition,* your blood pressure will be lower if you eat dark chocolate. At the Athens Medical School in Greece, subjects valiantly agreed to eat a 3.5-ounce bar of dark chocolate every day (think, 70% cocoa solids). Ultrasound tests of their blood vessels revealed an improvement in vessel wall flexibility for three hours following their consumption of the chocolate. Could follow-on studies then prove that chocolate can regulate blood pressure well enough to be part of a cardiac wellness program?

For a number of centuries, people have enjoyed chocolate. The Mayans valued it so much that they used cocoa beans as their currency. The Aztec Emperor Montezuma is said to have had as many as 50 cups a day of his preferred chocolate beverage. Thomas Jefferson thought chocolate must have superior qualities to tea or coffee. In this century, many agree that chocolate not only tastes good, it makes them somehow feel good. Can this be the instinct of good health?

Dr. Andrew Weil (*www.drweil.com*) suggests we limit ourselves to an ounce of very high quality dark chocolate (70% cocoa or more) several times a week. He recommends we enjoy quality over quantity to avoid the traps of excessive sugar, fats, and of course, calories. So enjoy your dark chocolate, and watch for future chocolate news!

# Relate From New Views

## Get Great Relationships with Three Top Tips

If you want the best energy, health, and wellness, take a fresh look at your relationships. Studies show that people with a network of supportive relationships are less likely to get serious medical conditions.

They are also more likely, if they do become ill, to become well. People with happy relationships are less prone to depression and more inclined to be financially successful. With satisfying relationships, people have a greater sense of well-being and simply enjoy life more.

So, do you want more satisfaction from the relationships you have? Do you want more close friendships? Do you perhaps have a business in which your client relationships could use some deepening? Would you like to reduce stress in conflicted relationships? If so, read on for the three top secrets of great relationships.

**The first secret of great relationships is to treat each person as though they are precious.** If you believe in a Divine Power, then you know the Divine holds each person to be precious, no matter how they look, sound, or act. Try to see each person as "a soul in a package." A person's physical form—their body, their appearance—is only packaging for the soul. In spare moments, practice imagining that you can see "the soul inside the package" of the people you see most often. Notice how you begin to care less about the externals you had been wishing they would change. Your teenager's pink hair will seem less important. Your neighbor's black lipstick and nails will fade in your awareness. That negative guy at the office will begin to seem less negative. When you truly treat another with respect, that is what you will get back. If someone speaks to you rudely, speak back as though they had spoken politely.

In situations with conflict, reply in a courteous, positive, interested manner. Most people will gradually shift, becoming polite and beginning to match your tone. You know this works in reverse. Many times, you have seen tones rise in anger, response by response, until a conversation has turned into a conflict. So now, with awareness, you can work it the opposite way to bring down dislike, disrespect, and conflict, notch by notch. If the relationship is already positive, you can deepen it with this method, as the person will absorb your respect more and more and reflect it back. Over time, this builds mutual trust and confidence. People will feel safe to express their minds and hearts around you.

**The second secret of great relationships is to listen to the other person's story.** Really listen. Make most of your conversation focus on the other person. Studies show that people crave to be loved, and the number one way that people feel they are loved is by others' listening to them. Ask questions, even if they sound initially superficial. During any holiday time, for example, you can turn to an acquaintance and ask, "So are there any foods you particularly like this time of year? Are there foods that really say 'Christmas' to you?" Then maintain eye contact and listen. What you will begin to hear is what is important to this person about the holidays, or what they find superficial and do not bother with at these times. You will begin to hear whether they do or don't get together with family or if they are closer with their friends than with their relatives.

Feel free to ask clarifying questions, since it shows the person that you really are listening and are interested. Ask "Wait, did you just say your sister comes from Ohio every year to ski in Flagstaff, Arizona? When there are tons of snow in Ohio? How did that get started?" Now you'll learn that ski slopes are much steeper in Arizona, and your friend prefers drinking espresso drinks while his sister is skiing the expert slopes. So the next time you meet your friend, meet him at a unique and charming espresso bar. Listening to others will get you out of your normal thought grooves and blow fresh ideas through your consciousness. You may find that, in getting to know them, you enjoy them more, and certainly they will feel closer to you because you inquired and listened.

**The third secret of great relationships is to make no assumptions.** Be open to who each person may really be. A person who is "messy" today may have stayed up all night with their ill parent at the hospital or with their asthmatic child at home. An "unfriendly" or "grumpy" person may be grieving. A "curt" person may be in physical pain. A "vague" person may need their other glasses, which are at home on the hall table. A "secretive" person may have a gossipy coworker who has previously damaged them with exaggerated careless whispers. You could be the first safe person these people have talked with in a long time.

Do not assume any unsmiling person needs cheering up and they need you to fix them! Do ask privately, with respect, and informally, "Are you OK?" Remember, others may be listening, so keep your voice down. If the person grumbles something back, ask quietly, "Can I help in any way?" At this point, they will probably say, "Oh, it's just my _____(back/4-year-old/Dad in hospital, car problem)." So now ask gently, "What's going on?" If they say they just want their space, and if you can honestly offer to listen at another time, say quietly, "Well, if you want talk later..." and now give them their space. Advice is completely unrequired in many situations, but your kindness will long be remembered and appreciated.

If someone begins to tell you all about their recent troubles, it is again not your personal mission to fix this person. Remembering that each person is precious, try to discern if the person just needs to vent. Do they just want to be heard, or do they want suggestions? If you can't clearly tell, ask, "Do you want any ideas on that?" If they don't want suggestions or help, just listen and then let them be.

Remember: each precious soul has a right to make choices along life's path. So if you want better, closer, deeper relationships, treat others with true respect, listen, and be open to who they are. In focusing on others, you will reap lifetime rewards.

## Love in Communication Styles

Do you want more love? People communicate respect, regard, caring, affection, and love in at least six different styles. When we know what some of these styles are, we suddenly notice the many, many signals of caring and love that are coming our way all the time. We can also then choose to get our love messages across in someone else's style, to be sure they're getting *our* signals.

The easiest ones to hear are *The Verbalizers*. They use words. They tell you "I love you," "You're super," "I'm so glad you're in my life," "We're so glad you could come for dinner this evening," "Let's get together again soon." You can use words back to them. This is clear. You know when these folks are expressing love.

Second easiest to understand are *The Gifters*. These folks show up with a flower from their garden, a packet of cookies they made, or a card for your birthday. Of course, they may bring fine chocolates and jewelry, and that's all right too. Some of these folks may even send you a plane ticket.

The third group is still somewhat easy to understand. These are *The Touchers*. They hug you hello, they touch your arm for emphasis, they hold your hand, they may rub your neck. They show they care through touch. One holiday, I went to join friends at their home. Their small nephew really likes people. As the front door opened, I saw a streak coming toward me. It was the Human Love Bullet! Little Riggs jetted into my leg, throwing his arms around my knee. I felt so loved.

The fourth type is often unrecognized. These are *The Do-Fors*. These people are always doing something for you. In men, this may take the form of always fixing things around your house. In women, this more often takes the form of cooking something for you or offering you something they have prepared. These folks bring your paper in from the driveway, pick up something you've dropped, and ask if you need anything from the grocery store. For a group, they volunteer to sing and do readings and prepare snacks for events.

Now, you may be thinking, "But, I give gifts *and* do things for people." Yes, you are a combination type. And most people are combination types. Your loved ones are lucky.

The fifth type is the most difficult love communicator for many people to understand. These are the *Quality Time People*. They hang out with you. They may call and just stay on the phone, and you're thinking, "What does this person want?" They're telling you they care about you by spending time with you. They may come by your house for no apparent reason. They want to spend time with you. *They* may not know this is their way of communicating regard, affection, or even love. But now *you* know. Plan activities with them. It may not matter what activity, just plan something, and spend time with them.

The last group is the *Cash Communicators*. They tell you they care with money. We see this in parents of college kids, who often ask, "How are things going? Do you need any money?" In this type of love communication, money is truly the currency of caring. Some people who can't communicate caring any other way rely on giving money as their means of sharing their love.

So we can see that love takes many forms. And there's so much more love going around than we have been recognizing. How about that kind driver on the freeway this week who sweetly pulled back to let you into the lane you needed? This is lovingkindness. How about the smile from a stranger in the grocery store? This is the look that tells you that another human wishes you well.

Love: it feels good and helps your health. Let's receive it, send it, and enjoy it, in all its forms. The Apostle Paul said, "Make love your aim." Now you can aim more accurately. And, now you can decode when love is aiming for you.

## Handle Hurtful People Effectively

On the opposite end of the relationship scale from love, we have difficult and destructive relating. Much has been written about dealing with difficult people, and this book will not attempt to summarize that extensive literature. However, it is vital to discuss the most hurtful people and the popular trap of making assumptions about values. When we assume others are operating from our values, we set ourselves up for surprises from those who enjoy hurting others.

As a "good person," I have often thought back to my childhood and other times and places in which my values were formed. I remember my mother talking about how we should live. I remember my father modeling the values Mother talked about, although he never discussed his philosophy.

My adult values are consciously based on my experience of the Divine and of the fundamental value of lovingkindness. I am aware of wanting to trust people, of wanting to be honest, of wanting to have goals based on my values, and of wanting to work in a focused way to achieve my goals. I am aware of wanting the best for others and for the world community, as well as the best for myself.

I believe there is no limit to goodness, and that everyone can be well, happy, and prosperous. I work hard to have a constructive lifestyle and to make a difference in relationships, in my community, and in the world. As a result of all this, I am who I am and have the lifestyle I have. I have many wonderful loving, fulfilling friendships and colleague- and client-relationships.

Not everyone operates according to my belief system. For example, many believe they can only have happiness or prosperity if they take it from someone else. In some, this is a reflex, not even a conscious thought set. These people will act differently than I do.

One of the greatest sources of negative stress is believing that events and people "should" operate in certain ways and then feeling bad when they don't. How many times have you listened to a friend for hours while they complained about the way someone else behaved? Think how bartenders must feel.

Have you ever been the one who moaned for hours over the behavior of a fellow student, a coworker, a neighbor, a famous person? How much energy did you spend wishing that person were different? How many times this week have you used the phrase "why don't you just…" or "why don't they just…"? That magic phrase tells you the speaker thinks s/he knows exactly how the person should behave. Notice how stressed the speaker sounds. With many people who are different from oneself, we need to simply affirm that they have a right to live their lives. They each have a right to their path.

However, there are times when someone else's behavior is very damaging to our reputation, our lifestyle, or our career. Then we must ask ourselves if philosophy and acceptance are enough, or if we need counseling, arbitration, a support group, a lawyer, or the police. Slander and libel are, respectively, the spoken and written untrue damaging claims that others make about us. These are major crimes because our justice system recognizes the extremely damaging nature of the actions. Stalking is the acting out of fascination with someone who doesn't want the attention. It is increasingly recognized by our justice system as criminal behavior with very damaging direct and indirect effects.

On a less obvious level, there is a range of ruthless and sociopathic behaviors that are damaging and difficult to counter. It may even be difficult to convince others the dynamics are occurring, depending on the intelligence and effective subtlety of the perpetrator. The solutions in this range are not simple. Fortunately, there are professionals who are exploring these extreme behaviors and publishing books about dealing with them.

Dr. Susan Forward writes about relationships with liars and manipulators. These people are frequently so clever that they can keep us believing that the problems they create are our fault. Try Dr. Forward's book, *Emotional Blackmail: When the People in Your Life Use Fear, Obligation, and Guilt to Manipulate You*. She has also written *Toxic Parents*; *Obsessive Love*; and *Men Who Hate Women and the Women Who Love Them*. Communications professor Jay Carter writes about difficult people, specifically those who will do anything at your expense. Look for his first book, *Nasty Men*, and his more comprehensive work, *Nasty People*. Are you dealing with someone who envies something about you, doesn't want what you have, but wants to take it away from you? Then try *The Sociopath Next Door* by Martha Stout.

Seek to understand your opponent and develop effective strategy, without wasting your time and energy on disbelief and anger. Stay focused on the best choices for your life. Remember, in the end, living well truly is the best revenge.

## Let Your Nature Nurture You

Not only can stress cause fatigue, but fatigue can cause stress. It's vital, if you are tired a lot, to ask yourself which started first. If you are ridiculously tired, one factor may be that you are forcing yourself to act against your true nature. This is incredibly wearing and leads to a lot of wasted energy, as well as misunderstandings in relationships.

Some people are even in a job or a profession that forces them to function against their true nature. In the classic American Winner Model, everyone is supposed to succeed by being forward, talkative, persuasive, and assertive. This is great for those whose temperaments are suited to this behavior, and it is very unhealthy for those who would be forcing themselves against type. Some people are trying to be quiet introverts working in cubicles away from other workers when they actually need interactive jobs surrounded by many persons and filled with ringing telephones. Others are trying to work in highly interactive environments that are giving them the sensation of being hammered; these workers need a quiet corner and a job structure with breakaway, stand-alone tasks. Some love to lead, and some love to follow. Some love to supervise and some love to sit doing repetitive tasks for years at a time. Fortunately, we need all these types in most work environments.

There are a number of useful personality inventory tests, and you may have taken several of them. I hope that you learned some interesting things about your nature from these systems. One useful framework that is not widely used is the oriental philosophy of the opposite natures, yin and yang. In Chinese philosophy, everything and everyone has a relatively yin or yang nature. Some substances and some people are very yang, and some are very yin.

Following is **Figure 7, Yin and Yang Characteristics**, illustrating the relative yin and yang of different qualities. See if one either yin or yang sounds more like the real you.

## Figure 7. Yin And Yang Characteristics

### YIN          YANG

| YIN | YANG |
|-----|------|
| Passive | Active |
| Weak | Strong |
| Cool | Warm |
| Dark | Light |
| Moon | Sun |
| Inward | Outward |
| Taking in | Giving forth |
| Left hand | Right hand |

### Feminine-Grounded          Masculine-Grounded

| Feminine-Grounded | Masculine-Grounded |
|-------------------|--------------------|
| Listening | Talking |
| Asking | Explaining |
| Responding | Initiating |
| "Taking in" | "Giving forth" |
| Nurturing | Caregiving |

If you like to express yourself verbally a lot during your work day or in your personal relationships, you may be more of a "yang-grounded" person. Try to be in jobs that require verbalizing, and find relationships with people who are listeners. Conversely, some of you are getting exhausted from the level of verbalizing required in your job and relationships. You have more of a "yin-grounded" nature, and it will always be exhausting to have to talk a lot. Try to be in jobs that can be handled with written communication and find a talker-initiator for your significant other.

Some of you are stressed out from supervising because you need to be in breakaway tasks (yin). Examine the possibilities for going down or across the organizational tree; you will spend less time and money on doctor visits. The more your life activities and your nature are in sync, the healthier, happier, and more peaceful you will be.

## Let Go of Advising

Now I want you to let go of something. How often have you heard someone ask, "Why don't you just…?" When someone is describing an uncomfortable situation in their life, especially at parties, many others think they wisely have a super solution. Often after hearing only a brief problem statement, and generally unasked, some people step forward with a little speech beginning "Why don't you just [do this to quickly solve it]?" This question is often asked in a tone of great frustration, as though it seems so obvious to the asker that, not only is there a quick solution, but they personally have the only one or the best one. But "knowing" what is best for others is illusory. One of the greatest sources of stress is worrying about what we can't control.

When we think that people should behave according to our plan and they behave differently, it generates frustration. In the extreme, it generates a sense of helplessness and sometimes depression. Physiologically, certain body circuits and organs reflect that frustration, and digestive biochemistry is commonly disrupted. When you are frustrated, eating fewer fats will ease your stress. Exercising helps.

Meditation helps. But the greatest strategy is to give up directing and advising others.

I invite you to give up, right now, wishing others would behave differently. I invite you to pause when you hear the words "Why don't you just…?" rising, and instead ask, "Do you want any suggestions?" If the person says "Well, yes!" then you're off and running in an interesting conversation. And you may have just the answers this person needs. However, if the person indicates they don't want suggestions, don't worry further. Just drop your shoulders, exhale, and let it go.

Don't absorb frustration into your body. Resolve to yourself to "love 'em where they're at," or chant silently "It is what it is." Their choices are not your problem. You are now in the next moment of your life. Let go of all your "shoulds" for others, and live your own life fully.

## Choose the B/Right Stuff

Words delightfully reflect how we look at things. One great example is the word "stuff." We speak of "owning stuff." We specify "that's my stuff, so leave it alone." We say, "I'm stuffed!" Some say, "Oh, stuff it!" In these phrases, we express ownership and stowage. In psychotherapy, the word "stuff" is used to mean one's emotional baggage, as in "all his stuff really came up in that argument." Psychological ownership and stowage come through in this usage, as in "stuffed emotions." In popular archetypes, our culture admires a hero who has "the right stuff," meaning that he is filled or "stuffed" with strong, positive traits that serve him and humanity well.

Would you like to size up your "stuff"? Then try the B/Right Stuff LifeTool. This is about making the bright choices and the right choices for your life. Do you have a notepad and pen or pencil? Let your imagination run free for a couple of minutes and try jotting down your answers to these questions for Part 1: What is important in life? What is right and what is wrong? What are your values? What is interesting? Do you run your life according to what is important to you? What is your "stuffing"? For your personal goals and values, do you have "the right stuff"? Is there a difference between what you say is right/important/interesting and what you spend your time on?

Now for Part 2, look around your living space briefly and keep writing, this time choosing adjectives for what you see. Do you see confusion, clutter, inconsistency, or incomplete projects? Does the air smell stagnant? Are there dirty or broken things or stuff that needs to be discarded? Right now, some of you are looking at a clean home, lovely colors, pretty furniture, clear walking spaces and exercise zones. Some of you have flourishing plants, clean air, and orderly files. All the food in your fridge is probably recognizable, and it's probably even fresh. Which home would you say has "the right stuff"? If you could move in now, which home would you choose?

For Part 3, work the process in reverse. How much do your descriptions of your "living space" match the "living space" of your mind? After all, bright people do much of their living in their minds. If your home needs dusting and cobweb removal, what about your thoughts? If some furniture is broken, what would it take to fix it? Then what would it take to repair the fixtures of your social life? If there is simply too much stuff in your home, are you often trying to deal with too many thoughts and activities in a week? How about reducing the "stuff" you cope with in your physical living and in your mental tasking? What can you "clean house" about? Can you drop an organization, leave one hobby to alternate years, or give a check instead of time to that fourth worthy cause?

Our homes are the outpicturing of our minds. How much clutter or gunk can be in the mind of a person with a clean, pleasant, and airy home? Just why do you think they call that one space a "living room"? Are you relaxed, happy, and satisfied in your mental living room? If not, here is an easy trick: clean your physical living room! Just as a cluttered mind generates a cluttered homescape, cleaning your homescape can clear your mind. Here's the really easy part: everything can be classified as either "Love It As Is" or "Other." The "Other" is of 3 types: "Clean It," "Fix It," and "Out, Out D—— Spot." If it's worth cleaning or fixing, do it; hire a little help if you need to. Otherwise, toss it or donate it.

Now, what's in your house? Write that down. Do you see a pattern? When we get rid of the Wrong Stuff, we end up with only the Right Stuff. After this exercise, notice how many nice new people you meet in the following two weeks. Notice how your mind is clearer and your goals are starting to take orderly mental form. Notice how you're more effective in the workplace and in social groups. Your former resistance to cleaning up your "stuff" was holding you back on many levels.

Hey, now that you've "cleaned house" with your living room, have you thought about "straightening out" your "bedroom stuff"? Wow! Think of the possibilities and write them down. Clear the Wrong Stuff from the rooms of your physical house and the Right Stuff will express in many ways in your lifestyle. Make the b/right choices for you. Enjoy choosing your stuff and your life, starting now.

## Stump Your Stale-O-Meter<sup>sm</sup> with Microshift

In music, the "upbeat" creates uplift in each measure. A key part of my mission is to draw attention to the "Up Beat" of life, the positive areas and potentials of lifestyle. If you have been feeling the need for a bit of uplift, perhaps this section is for you.

Have things seemed a bit flat lately? I have long taught the naturalness of change. All processes result in change, in shift. Many say, "Shift happens." Others say, "We make shift happen." I say, "Microshift creates uplift."

Much has been written about change and how people tend to fear large-scale change. However, some small forms of change delight us. When our baby learns a new sound or motor skill, we feel a rush of joy. We may burst out laughing and call someone in from the next room to share the delight. A cool, rainy day can make us smile after years of drought and months of heat. A "change of scene" can refresh us as we take a vacation after months of nonstop work and local routine. New information can cause inspiration. Just the intake of new ideas can change the way we view people, life, and the world. Some microshift is caused by our choices, and some is included in our thoughts through observation.

Do you want to experiment? How bored, stuck, or stale do you feel right now? Pick your own scale, such as the "Stale-o-meter," where "ten" is feeling completely stale, bored, stagnant, or flat and "zero" is feeling totally vital, refreshed, stimulated, inspired, and generally excited with life. On the scale you've picked, write down your self-score for your current state. Now offer your mind some microshift as you consider some of the new phenomena in different aspects of life.

1.  The Smithsonian Institute, once only a site to visit in Washington, D.C., now has Culturefest programs around the country. The Smithsonian Associates now take cultural and scientific treasures on tour with speakers and concert presentations.
2.  There is now a science of fragrance and flavor generation. The City Museum of Stockholm recently had a British scientist create a "disgusting" odor for an exhibit on ancient medicines featuring mummification. In British nursing homes, a fragrance called "granny's kitchen" and one called "coal fire" are used therapeutically to assist elderly dementia patients.
3.  In Florida and the Caribbean, after recent hurricanes, there have been ecosystem shifts. These have resulted in a population explosion for the spadefoot toad, with many millions of baby spadefoot toadlets now hopping around the landscape.
4.  In the world of wine, the next oenophile horizon is Geneva—yes, Geneva, Switzerland. While only 1% of the annual wine output of Switzerland gets exported, a target market has recently been found in Brussels, since Belgium is too cold for growing grapes.
5.  In Dubai, the United Arab Emirates, the temperature often gets to 130 degrees Fahrenheit. An indoor Alpine-skiing facility has been built, attached to a major shopping mall, by an international team.
6.  The newest "green" textiles are made from bamboo. Not only can you buy bamboo flooring, you can now purchase pillows and fashions made from bamboo fiber.

So, now how is your Stale-o-meter self-score? I hope that, after looking at novel information, it is noticeably lower. This is "microshift," tiny changes created with little time, effort, or cost. What would happen

if you actually did something different today? Call an old friend, try a
new friend, visit a new restaurant, or order a different dish. See a movie
someone else picked. Plan a vacation or conference trip. Just thinking
out the details will refresh your mind, whether or not you actually go.

Join a special interest organization. Clean out a closet and take the
extras to a charity. Visit a new church or local meetings of a political
party. Go to a lecture, an art opening, or a student concert. Volunteer to
serve at a soup kitchen, to work in a food bank, or to deliver senior
lunches. Inquire about having your dog trained as a therapy dog. Offer a
course at a senior center or community college. Invite a few people over
to watch a provocative film, fiction or documentary. Thinking about this
list, has your Stale-o-meter score shifted? Are you perhaps feeling more
energized?

If not, consider changing your input sources and settings. Novelty
stimulates. Try Microshift for Uplift$^{sm}$, daily for seven days, and check
your Stale-o-meter again. If you're enjoying yourself so much that you
forget to note your Stale-o-meter score, it's definitely working. We need
shift, and we can make shift happen. The quality of your life depends on
you. Why not choose the greatest quality now?

## Manage Your Moods With Energy Balancing

We may sometimes realize that we have physical discomforts which are
related to stress and emotional burdens. From fatigue and appetite
problems to skin eruptions and ulcers, our bodies may store our
distressful experiences. Spiritual, mental, and emotional ills can make us
feel bad physically. Also, if we feel bad physically, it is harder to feel
great emotionally, mentally, and spiritually.

There are many easy physical techniques to help ourselves shake off/let
go of/release stress, and the following sections cover major groups of
these. You are about to learn simple, portable LifeTools to help you
center yourself, loosen up, energize, or release, including release of
pain.
Finger holds and pressure points are related to acupressure, the art of
using access points to the nervous system to release build-ups of
discomforts.

## Center and Find Stillness

When we quiet the busy body we can quiet the busy mind. The more still we are outside, the more we can find that quiet space inside our hearts and spirits. The more quietude we can experience, the more we can hear the "little voice" inside which is really the "Big Voice", the Voice of God, Kol Adonai (Hebrew for Voice of God), or the Christ-Self. The more we practice getting in touch with our innermost selves when we are physically still, the easier it becomes to start carrying the sure Quiet around in externally chaotic times.

Try this LifeTool for centering. Gently allow your shoulders to drop. Place your center three fingertips of each hand in the center of each opposite palm. Hold at least three to five minutes. Feel the metabolism slow and any trembling melt away.

## Loosen Up

When we have tension, the body gets tight in ways and places we don't always notice quickly. We have much more energy when we loosen the tightness and let our natural miraculous energy, blood, oxygen, lymph service, and good feelings flow.

Try this LifeTool for loosening up. Stand, then "S-E-L-F": Shrug, Exhale, Laugh, Feel the difference. Do this at different speeds to feel the effects. The shrugs must be smooth, stretching, gentle, and slow. Avoid making sudden or jerky moves.

Try this additional LifeTool for loosening the body system. Put on an uplifting piece of music and slowly shrug every way you can think of for two minutes. Now extend "shrugging" to the equivalent for the arms, hands, legs, feet, abdomen. Experiment. Again, use smooth, gentle movements. The benefits are in the "going," not the "getting there."

Energize

Now that you have practiced centering and loosening, let's power up.
Let's release the body's natural vigor. Try this LifeTool for energizing.
Place your hands together in a "praying hands" position. Feel the energy
between the hands. Fold the fingers together. Hold this position for at
least five minutes and feel the energy all over the body. Now you know
why prayer positions for hands are so popular.

Release

Releasing stress and pain feels good and means less effort is required to
live each hour. It takes more work to hold in pain and hurts than it does
to release them.

Try these three LifeTools for rapid releasing.

First, gently hold and take three complete breaths on each finger and
then the palm center. Start by gently grasping your left thumb with your
right hand. Wrap the right fingers and thumb around your left thumb as
if "hugging" it. Don't squeeze. Pressure is not necessary or helpful.
Take 3 slow, complete breaths and move to holding your left forefinger.
Repeat with each finger on both hands. Also, touch your right fingertips
to the left palm and take 3 slow, complete breaths, then repeat with the
left fingertips to the right palm.

Second, hold the thumb-forefinger web about an inch below the large
knuckle of the forefinger. Hold the muscle that feels like firm tofu. This
is a general pain releaser for the body.

Third, place the thumb of each hand over the ring-fingernail of the same
hand, and hold as long as you like. This releases constricted breath or
lessens temporary pain, such as that caused by dental drilling.

# Discharge Strong Negativity

At times in life, we experience very strong negative feelings. One of the most uncomfortable, and often damaging, emotions is anger. It comes in the guise of impatience, resentment, jealousy, frustration, and even violence. Much has been written on the psychology, derivation, interactions, and effects of anger. There are books on assertiveness and books on dialoguing. But when can you use all that information? Analysis and dialoguing are wonderful for understanding your anger and getting clear on what you would like to communicate.

But what if you literally can't talk with the one you're angry with, such as a particular person, an entity, or a societal issue? The particular person (Mom, a romantic partner, a professor, an attacker) may have died, or perhaps you have no way to contact them. Perhaps it is inappropriate or highly risky to express anger to your boss. Perhaps the parent you feel anger toward, if still living, is too ill for you to talk with. Perhaps that former spouse has moved away to an unknown location.

The entity (The Rich, General Motors, The Government, Dishonest Businesspeople) may be difficult to contact by its size, multiple locations, or diffused structure. And it's hard to speak your anger directly to a societal issue (abortion rights, street violence, education opportunities, zoning requirements, gang activities, feeding the hungry, global environments) because they are never at their desks for appointments.

When the object of your strong negativity is unavailable, and you must deal with your feelings yourself, try these practical and satisfying approaches to discharging your feelings.

1. **Write it.** Write a searing letter saying whatever you think/feel in whatever language. Ball it up, throw it all over the room, stomp on it. Burn it in a very safe fireproof place (be careful: it will flame high).

2. **Change your expectations** of the person/entity. You can change only you, not them.

3. **Know that the past was a giant workshop.** If the anger has to do with an abusive past, realize that the deep unhappiness of the past is the finest foundation for savoring the wonderful life you are now creating for yourself.

4. **Allow yourself constructive rebellion.** Go to the park during lunch, or take an afternoon off from work. Be yourself. Get a new hairstyle, bright clothes, that sports car, or start wearing hats. Do things differently today.

5. **Release by pounding soft things.** Grab a pillow and pound on a couch or an easy chair. With your fists, pound a *padded* carpet or a mattress.

6. **Tell it to the empty chair**. Preferably with a professional facilitator present, imagine the person or entity present in an empty chair you have chosen. Tell them exactly what you think and call them anything you want. Be perfectly honest. Scream and cry if you want to. You are not done until you feel bored! Now order the person to leave and visualize them going out the door, never to disturb your happiness again. Do it again anytime you feel it would be satisfying.

7. **Scream** Shout into a pillow until you are tired of it. This is satisfying, and no one can hear it!

8. **Smash junk.** Having saved some cheap dishes for the purpose, smash them on a concrete walk or garage floor. Throw them down hard. Choose your location! This can sound like someone smashing a windshield and you may get attention you don't want, which is no fun when you are this upset.

9. **Pound things with a bataca.** Pound any stuffed furniture with a bataca, a padded tool with a handle made for exactly this.

10. **Crash your books.** If they are your books and you feel like it, pull all of them off the bookcase rapidly. The downsides are that someone has to pick them up and they may get damaged.

11. **Stamp on paper towels.** Take an unopened roll, and throw it around, pound it, stamp on it. Throw it to the floor very hard. You can still use all the paper towels later, since they are clean.

12. **Clean, clean, clean!** Play super-cleaner and scrub every speck of dirt, dust, and grime out of those floors, cupboards, and tiles. Do as much as you can until you are exhausted. This is great for venting. It gives a satisfying feeling with lovely and healthy results.

13. **Throw ice.** Get a lot of ice cubes and throw them against a concrete wall as hard as you can. They make a lovely shattering sound. Imagine each one to be whatever issue or person you like.

Repeat any of these until you are bored. Now you are done discharging. But would you like a more profound release?

Then get revenge by joy. **Living well is the very best revenge!** Create success for yourself, including happy, loving relationships. "Show them" by being happy, healthy, well-groomed, prosperous, and loved. You may even convert their attitude, by example, through yours.

## Manage Burnout and Energy Emergencies

**If you are even thinking of the word "burnout," you are in burnout. Follow the list below for three days, while you consider major changes.** Then, go back to the beginning of this book and work your way through, making notes and developing your new plan for your life-energy management.

**Immediately, you must:**

1. Drink a large mug or glass of filtered water.

2. Sit down.

3.  Exhale to the end of your breath and allow a reflexive inhale. Do this twice more.

4.  Determine how soon you can get to a quiet place for ten minutes and do it as fast as you can. This may be your car in the parking garage.

5.  Breathe quietly for ten minutes, thinking of quiet, peace, serenity, and strength. If you are a spiritual person, think of your Divine Source. After about ten minutes, think of how wonderfully and easily you focus.

**Within the next three days, you must:**

1.  Switch to eating mainly fresh, raw fruits and vegetables. Also emphasize cooked nonstarchy vegetables, such as those found in stir-fry recipes.

2.  Put some sesame seeds in a small container in your desk, your car, your pocket. Toss a teaspoon or so of these in your mouth and chew well several times a day. These will yangize your metabolism, strengthening you and clearing your mind. You can get sesame seeds in the spice section of any grocery store, or in bulk at many health food stores.

3.  Get some Bach Rescue Remedy (naturopathic stress-relief drops) from a large health-food store, and take it several times per day. Follow the label for dosage.

4.  Take a few minutes to rise and stretch every hour.

5.  Exhale completely and drop your shoulders whenever you think of it.

6.  Make a list of everything you are grateful for, from your cat and your favorite grooming items to nice people, clouds, and God.

7.  Find a professional therapist or a coach to help see you through this time and see them at their next open appointment. Tell your

co-workers and family you have a can't-miss doctor's appointment. Make no excuses. Go.

8.  Check your sleep habits and get an herbal sleep remedy from a health-food store if you need it. A good one is Rescue Sleep, from the Bach Flower Remedies line. Do not drink alcohol or eat sugared foods before bed. Warm chamomile or mint tea an hour before bedtime may help you.

9.  Ask yourself what you need to change and start a list. Begin working with your doctor or other professional to determine how you will change it to get out of this condition and stay balanced for the long term.

## Get Professional Bodywork/Energy Therapy

Do you have a health concern or find yourself feeling "stressed out"? Do you want some type of treatment you may not have tried before, either to solve a specific body discomfort or to "just relax" and "get the stress out"? There is a wonderland caring professionals offering to help you feel better. Many options are open to you. Why not experiment?

Bodywork therapies range from pure *massotherapy* (hands manipulating your skin/muscles/fascia) to pure energy work (direct energy conveyance, therapist's hands need not actually contact your skin). Massotherapy varies from very light to very deep and from general to specific. Energy work without massotherapy is gentle to your tissues and varies from general (such as a basic *Reiki* treatment) to specific (such as a Jin Shin Jyutsu treatment). Many modalities (types or classes of therapy) combine massotherapy and energy work. Some therapists combine more than one modality in a session. Each system and each therapist is perfect for some people. How, then, do you decide which kind(s) of therapy may be just right for you?

First, think about what you most want to address. Is it an arm or a leg or a muscle group that has gradually stiffened for no apparent reason? Is it a specific pain or an area that never really recovered after an accident? Is it a general feeling of tightness or fatigue that is with you a lot now while your life is frustrating/grieving/extra busy? Different therapy modalities have different characteristics and strengths. Check the brief descriptions below and see which experience sounds most appealing to try. Later, you may like to try others also, and compare what works for you. Following are some of the common modalities presently available.

### Massotherapy

Massotherapy, or *massage therapy*, always moves the tissues and generally requires the client to undress, then be draped over any body areas that are not being worked at the moment. Following are some popular types of massage therapy.

*Swedish Massage*:  Traditional stress-release therapeutic massage using mostly smooth gliding movements with lotion. This can be light to deep. Component movements include gliding, kneading, vibration, range-of-motion (joint mobility), and percussion. It is generally soothing and calming. Note: "Full body massage" excludes the groin and female breasts in most jurisdictions. See below on "Dressing and Draping."

*Deep Muscle Therapy*:  Deeper therapy to release muscular pain problems and joint immobility problems due to muscular or myofascial stiffness. This is done with or without lotion depending on areas to be addressed and type of tightness. When appropriate, this may be done vigorously with rock music or other high-energy music playing.

*Rolfing*:  Deep tissue therapy, often recommended as a series of ten sequential treatments. A system designed by Ida Rolf, its practice may include techniques similar to deep muscle therapy, together with evaluation of posture and body movement for more effective athletic performance or relief of discomforts. Rolfing emphasizes release of inappropriate tissue attachments and "restructuring" of previously "stuck" body zones. Rolfers may have a separate professional certification (Certified Rolfer) or license, depending on the jurisdiction.

*Sports Massage*:  This is offered by therapists specifically oriented to solving the problems of people active in sports and body training.

Usually deep muscle therapy, with or without lotion, depending on the nature and location of the discomfort to be addressed.

*Integrated Neuromuscular Therapy*: Very specific myofascial therapy for extremely tight areas, such as the neck that cannot be turned in the morning. Movements use little or no lotion. Movements feel light to moderate, yet affect tissues which are very deep, resulting in a thorough clearing of muscular and myofascial tightness.

## Combination Therapies

*Acupuncture*: Energy therapy often utilizing special needles (thus having physical impact and making it a combination technique) to contact nervous system access points. This is used by the Chinese Army for a variety of health adjustments, as these needles can be applied through clothing. If you don't like needles, *accupressure* uses the same points without them. [Note: "acu" is from the root word for "needle," so accupressurists often use "accu" from "accurate" instead. This is why you'll see spelling variations.] Acupuncture is a cluster of related disciplines, and needle appearance and practice will vary.

*Foot Reflexology*: Massage/accupressure technique done with the client fully clothed, socks off. This practice is based on the idea that the nerves for the entire body can be reached reflexively through the feet. It relaxes, energizes, and balances the whole being. It may be applied as primarily massotherapy, as primarily index-accupressure (with a foot reflex diagram used as an index map of the body), or as a combination of the two.

*Reflexology*: Usually meaning foot reflexology, as above. May also mean *facial reflexology* (using a face reflex diagram as an index map of the body), *hand reflexology* (you guessed it), or *ear reflexology* (such as pulse reading for determining substance sensitivities). Some use the word to mean all classes of reflexology, or the practice of harmonizing portions of the body from other parts of the body through nervous-system reflexes. Whole-body reflexology is done through such methods as *Jin Shin* (Jyutsu or Do) or generic accupressure. Facial reflexology may be used in combination with facial toning for beauty, relaxation, or harmonizing goals.

*Shiatsu* and *Tui Na*:  Each a great art in its own right, both Shiatsu (Japanese) and Tui Na (Taoist Chinese) combine a variety of massotherapy strokes and pressures with progression along energy meridians to achieve releases. Each can be general or specific, as you request. The client is generally fully clothed for these treatments.


## Energy Therapy

*Jin Shin Jyutsu/Accupressure*:  Specific energy technique done with client fully clothed. Pairs of points along energy meridians are held in specific sequences to "jumper cable" the body energy back into balance. Great for "tuning up," relaxing and releasing stress, addressing headaches and other discomforts. Jin Shin Do is another form of this.

*Reiki*:  Energy technique done with client fully clothed. It looks like "laying on of hands," as the hands are placed in pairs on twelve or more key body energy centers. This energizes and balances the whole being and brightens mood. Specific hand positions may be added to the base treatment to give certain body zones extra attention. This can be done as *Christian Reiki*, with emphasis on Christian healing concepts.


## Choosing Your Therapist

It is key to your feeling-good/harmonizing/healing process to be comfortable with your therapist. Would you be more comfortable with a female therapist or with a male therapist? Then keep this in mind, especially if you have not had bodywork before. Your first experience should ideally open a window to many wonderful experiences of release and relaxation.

Call the therapist with whom you are considering scheduling an appointment. Ask that individual, not the receptionist, about any concerns you may have at this time. Some offices have printed information they would be delighted to mail or email to you. Also, you

can visit most clinics/treatment offices/salons ahead of time and see the
treatment room (between their appointments, of course) and its
environment. If you are uncomfortable, ask questions or go on to the
next place on your list.

### Points To Consider

1. Music/environment:  Do you like a quiet environment? Massage in
   a salon with rock music coming through the walls may not be for
   you. Or it may be perfect if you like a high-energy deep muscle
   therapy session. Each therapist creates her/his own setting, often
   through the use of quiet lighting and peaceful music. Some use
   pastel or other color groupings to help you relax visually from the
   moment you enter.

2. Talking:  Do you enjoy talking out your discomforts or relaxing into
   a "melted" mass while the therapist works? Ask if the therapist likes
   to work in your mode.

3. Fees/time:  An hour is a typical length of a treatment session,
   although less or more may be best for some people. Ask not only
   what the hourly fee is but how far apart appointments are scheduled.
   If appointments are always booked on the hour, your "hour" of
   therapy will allow about fifty minutes of therapy time. If one-hour
   appointments are booked every hour-and-a-quarter, you will have
   sixty minutes of therapy time. So take care in comparing prices "per
   hour." In some offices, new clients have an additional consultation
   just prior to the first treatment; this assures that the therapist can
   fully understand the client's health background and goals.

4. Skin/breathing sensitivities:  If your skin reacts badly to oil, specific
   oils, certain lotion ingredients, or fragrances, ask if this therapist can
   or does work without these. In therapy rooms adjacent to perming or
   nail care stations, chemical odors may enter. If you are sensitive to
   such odors, check the room before committing to an appointment.
   That location may or may not work for you.

## During Your Appointment

1.  Dressing and Draping:  For massotherapies, some undressing is usually required. Most jurisdictions require draping of the body, and most therapists carefully drape all portions of the body not being treated at that moment.

2.  Comfort Zones:  At any time during your session, if you are uncomfortable, tell the therapist. Hands can massage with less pressure, music volume can be lowered, and rooms can usually be warmed. Unusual physical sensations can be corrected (i.e., energy stream "zings" or your knee being stretched too far). Therapeutic discomfort is different from pain. If you are uncomfortable with the therapist's behavior, feel free to stop the treatment. This person or this therapy may not be for you.

## After Your Appointment

If your therapist recommends that you do some support activities for yourself between treatments, do try these suggestions! These self-helps may range from mild stretching exercises to hot soaks to holding an accupressure point or two. Doing these activities for a few minutes a day can promote your harmonizing process, reduce discomforts, and increase your energy and joy. May your explorations in the world of therapy be both satisfying and fun!

# Reflections

# Chapter 4

# RISE HIGHER

Within each of us is a spiritual dimension that needs to be nurtured for each to fully Discover The Secret Energized You. Each of us needs to determine our beliefs about the Divine and our spiritual role in the Universe. From those beliefs, each person's personal spiritual practice will develop. Some will pray, some will meditate, some will walk in natural settings, and some will go to houses of worship. This chapter includes four LifeTools sets for the spiritual side of your grand experiment: Life. How high will your spiritual life rise? Let it truly empower and uplift you.

> **There are only two ways to live your life.
> One is as though nothing is a miracle.
> The other is as though everything is a miracle.
> —Albert Einstein**

## Forgive

When I was a child, I sometimes heard the phrase "forgive and forget." I often puzzled over this phrase. It seemed to basically mean "set aside others' meanness as though it didn't happen." In those years, I knew people who enjoyed being angry and holding resentment. It was as if the ability to blame someone else, young or grown, for being out of line, actually empowered the one feeling resentment. When I was small, the most practical reason I could see for letting go of someone else's bad behavior or communication was to prevent the escalation of heated words into dangerous violence. A practical child was I, with a useful philosophy for being around volatile adults.

Psychologically, when you walk around resenting others, you are carrying a burden. A cleric I knew liked to ask, "How many people have you brought to church with you who don't even know they're here?"

Medical science of recent decades has proven out much folk wisdom. We now know it is wise to forgive, and holding onto negativity hurts only the one who feels negative. It is hazardous to your health and physical comfort to hold onto anger and resentment. Every emotion causes specific biochemistry in the body, and certain body systems are likely to fail first when resentments are held. Some people have released terribly crippling painful conditions when they released the emotions, and therefore the biochemistry, of resentment and anger. They literally stopped holding these negative emotions inside.

Still, what is "forgiveness," and how can you do it? Many have said, "Oh, be the better person and apologize for the argument, and then all will be forgiven." This is the technique I call "The Agreed Re-set$^{sm}$." It is probably the most commonly attempted way of "forgiving." It is basically like my childhood technique, a choice to "forget" and act as though a conflict or injury had not occurred. However, this technique can leave a lot of feelings and biochemical compounds buried deep in your system.

A better technique is the LifeTool I call the "Seventy Times Seven Release$^{sm}$." Here, you write "I forgive_____" seventy times every day for seven days. You will be amazed at how powerful this technique is. You'll need to start with several pencils or pens, since one or more will malfunction as you begin. You agree in advance not to let your hand leave the paper until all seventy statements are on the page. You will feel many body sensations during this exercise, but stick with it for the rewards.

By the end of the week, you'll feel not only physically different, but also emotionally different towards the object of resentment, only vaguely remembering what the issue ever was. This technique works because of Neuro-Linguistic Programming principles which dovetail with Christian principles. Jesus advised his followers to forgive "seventy times seven."

# Connect

The more fluently, deeply, and completely you can connect with the Divine, the more you will experience the miraculous levels of

The Secret Energized You. You can actually experience more miracles! So how can you increase your connection?

The Divine has many names, among them God, Yahweh, Jehovah, Spirit, The Universe, Limitless Intelligence, Upstairs Management, and "Help!" As a minister, I don't really care what you call God, as long as you call God. So what is God's phone number? I'll get to that, so have your pen ready.

It has been said that many people want to serve the Divine but mostly in a purely advisory capacity. Many people talk *to* Heaven/God/Angels/Spirit/The Universe/Limitless Intelligence, especially to say what they want and what they want the Divine to do. They give Heaven's staff their shopping lists for relationships, conditions, and possessions.

However, what is happening in the other half of the conversation? How does the Divine talk with us, or try to? Here are four top categories of communication from The Universe—and these are not all the possible forms there are. As I describe these, I believe many of you will begin to remember stories of similar occurrences from your own life, and I strongly encourage you to make notes and journal them out later or discuss them with a friend. There are technical names for some of these phenomena, but I invite everyone to be open to fresh thoughts about the occurrences I'm describing. Here's a chance for some new perspective.

> **When the gods come among men,**
> **they are not known.**
> **—Ralph Waldo Emerson**

The first form of communication from the Divine often slips right by people. *It's when you know something you don't know.* In college days, I began to realize that, as I approached a telephone to call someone, I knew whether they would be answering before I even picked up the receiver. When this happens, you are hooked into the pool of Limitless Intelligence, and you are accessing the Universal database. You know something you have no *earthly* way of knowing.

The second form of communication from Spirit I call *urges with miraculous effect*s. As a college kid, I was driving a friend through a sleepy small town. We stopped at a red light, and the cross-traffic was one-way, coming from our right. When the light turned green, the cross-traffic was perfectly clear. Oddly, though, I had a strong sensation to just wait a moment. Out of nowhere, a car appeared from our right, flying double speed! Had I not waited, my friend would have been crushed, and I probably wouldn't be here either. We were both shocked and very impressed. I had received an urgent nonverbal communication that very clearly said, "WAIT!" although I didn't actually hear the word "wait." Were my friend and I glad I was listening, as Spirit was communicating?

One year I was doing some work in rural Arizona, and I was up on a hill, waiting for a colleague to meet me. While I was waiting, I started taking photographs of the cactus and scenery. I was backing up to get just the right angle on a blooming ocotillo when suddenly every fiber of my body yelled "STOP!" It wasn't a word, but an urge, an imperative kinesthetic message to freeze. I froze. I looked behind me, and a few inches from my back boot heel was an unmarked open vertical mine shaft. I eased away from it, and after I recovered from the shock a bit, I tossed a stone down the shaft. The shaft was probably 200 feet deep, or more. An urge saved my life. Am I glad I was listening?

A third form of communication from the Divine is *hearing someone who isn't there, or seeing them, or hearing and seeing them.* This may be a communication from Heaven at a time when you are being asked to serve. My biggest service of this kind, so far, was one that evolved when I was visiting a B&B in a small town.

I was the only guest at breakfast, and I became aware of someone to my right trying to get my attention. And he seemed to be in a wheelchair. I was extremely hungry, so I tried saying, "I'm trying to eat breakfast here—can't this wait?" But what he wanted was for me to translate some information from him to the B&B owner, who was serving breakfast but likely to leave shortly. He said who he was, and I recognized his name. I knew he was the B&B owner's friend who had died a few weeks before. So I found a way to introduce the conversation, and we carried on a 3-way communication for nearly an hour.

My wheelchair-bound visitor wanted his friend to know he had not died the way she thought he had. Rather, he said, he had died the way he wanted to. He was emphatic that she should not feel guilty, since he was joyful over the way he had died. This conversation was nothing short of miraculous. It provided great relief to the B&B owner, who had thought she was, in part, responsible for her friend's death. It was a great joy to be of service to them.

When I went upstairs to rest, exhausted, my visitor followed me, thanking me effusively. I asked him, "Why did you pick me? I knew your name, and I knew you were her great friend, but I had never met you." He said, "That's exactly why I wanted you, for the communication to be credible." Now, am I glad I was willing to listen? Would you be willing to listen ... and serve?

The last major type of Divine communication is that of *unreasonable manifestations, often through the animal kingdom.* Some simply call these "miracles." But let us not allow that word "miracles" to sidetrack us from the fact of God in action in these scenes. You may remember that, a couple of years ago, a small child fell into a gorilla enclosure at an environmental zoo. The lead gorilla cradled the injured child until other humans could come to help her. That gorilla was tuned in to the Divine frequency and was serving.

Another powerful example of unreasonable manifestation occurred in Ethiopia. A girl had been beaten and was bleeding as she fled her village. Three lions appeared, held the attackers at bay, and protected the girl until the police came. Then they let the police help her. Not only did the lions not eat the girl for lunch, they discerned which humans had helpful intentions and which had violent intentions toward the girl. Only the Divine could put lions to work, protecting a bleeding girl.

There are a number of ways the Divine could have caused this scene. The lions may have been guided by Holy Spirit, Divine Intelligence. Or they may have been Angels or Spirit Guides who embodied only long enough to save the girl and make the international news. It is important to note that the international wire services covered this story—because this girl's attack was part of a larger problem that needs to be aired out by public outrage and public prayer. Perhaps God was using the girl and the lions to publicize internationally the need for the end of ethnic violence.

On the light side, there is a classic joke about people's expectations of God/Spirit/The Divine/Limitless Intelligence: A town is being flooded, and a boat comes by the home of man named "John". The firemen urge John to get in the boat with his dog and be saved. John says, "No, thank you, God is going to save me!" Another boat comes by, and now the water is up to the second floor. Again, John declines, saying God will save him. The floodwaters continue to rise. John and his dog are on the roof, and a helicopter comes by, the crew offering to save John and the dog. Yet again, John declines, saying God will save him. John and his dog drown. They arrive at Heaven Main Office, and John is frustrated! He says to God, "God, why didn't you save me?" And God answers, "John, I sent you two boats and a helicopter!" John's prayers and faith were answered in forms other than what he was expecting, and he rejected the answers. How many times have you prayed and rejected the response?

So what is God's phone number? If you're ready to step up and phone up and listen up, dial I-L-I-S-T-E-N! Pick a quiet place. Spend ten to twenty minutes at a time just listening or meditating. Make notes and journal. Pray, certainly, in the style you prefer. Or simply set your intention to hear what you most need to hear. Then listen again, observe, make notes, journal. Notice the new and the miraculous occurring in your relationships, your health, your joy, and your finances. Get into a closer relationship with Spirit—and not just in an advisory capacity. The Divine can take you places you've only ever dreamed of!

## Change With Change

Would you believe traffic is terrifically congested in Hawaii, and development is increasingly reducing the native feel of the islands? In a Charlie Chan novel set near Honolulu, the characters comment on this—in 1918. Would you believe, "We live in a time of very great change"? You might say, "Well, duhhhhh!" Yet this quote is from Britain's Queen Victoria in 1861. Change is a normal part of human experience. Yet many people fight change and feel stressed by it. They get fatigued thinking wistfully of the way things used to be. Wouldn't you have more energy if you embraced change or even let the possibilities excite you?

Recent years have been times of exponentially increasing change. As we rolled into the year 2000, Millennium commentators cited many examples of technological, economic, and social change during the twentieth century. On December 31, 1999, CNN cameras showed public celebrations with fireworks near the White House, the Eiffel Tower, and the Pyramids.

When the White House and the Eiffel Tower were designed, each was debated as a drastic departure from the architecture of the time. One was thought too plain for its purpose, and the other too stark and ugly. Each, in its time, was regarded as representing too much change. Yet each is now a beloved symbol. I suspect that the Pyramids may have been hotly debated in their time, too. Yet they now stand among the greatest architectural achievements of humankind. One of the truths of humanity is that we accustom ourselves to change.

Throughout human history, people and countries have eventually adapted to the results of invasions, wars, plagues, natural disasters, population migrations, economic shifts, and technological change. For each person, there is surprise, shock, grief, sometimes anger, sometimes denial, and eventually, acceptance of each change. As individuals and countries, we ask ourselves how we want things to be and how we can best get there. We then assess what resources we bring to a situation, and we apply those as best we can.

I wrote a column on September 11, 2001, as the World Trade Center and the Pentagon had just been attacked. The skies were suddenly made silent, and in that silence our thinking changed forever. While we saw the ugliest, angriest sides of human nature in those attacks, we also saw massive kindness, caring, and service to others blossoming everywhere. That week, it seemed that everyone was looking at everyone else with new eyes—huge, hurt, inquiring eyes. Many people became more aware of the beliefs, ethnicities, and national origins of those around them. I noticed more attentiveness, even in traffic. Some of us cried for weeks.

In the years since the attacks, we have seen cultural, practical, and economic shifts. It has become wonderful rather than corny to love this country and display our flag. It has become normal, not "dorky," to speak admiringly of firefighters, police, and military veterans. It has become normal for men to speak of strong feelings and shed tears. It is common to travel less by air, pack less, and expect longer lines for airport security. War movies of all eras are back. It is normal now to celebrate our freedom and talk about global peace. We have been adjusting, as individuals, as peoples, as countries, and as a planet united in active dialogue. An adage from timeless wisdom advises "Nothing stays the same but change."

Whatever your belief system, you can be a part of the world's next set of positive changes. Golda Meir said, "Anyone who thinks one person can't make a difference... has never been to bed with a mosquito." So why not drop your shoulders and exhale the past? Will you change with change and step eagerly into your future? It's up to you.

## Carpe Diem, Not the Fish of the Day

I had a friend who managed all the computer systems for an Army base. The work was interesting, the pay was excellent, and Ginny was treated well. The catch was that she was on call 24 hours a day, most days of the year. Sometimes it really added up, and she could get massively tired and crabby. She could have complained, but she had a heavenly stress antidote. She went fishing twice a year, out of pager range. At least, that's what she claimed to do. One year, she told me the real secret: this was her chance to just sit still, for several days, away from phones. Ginny had learned to trade carping for trout.

Another friend of mine owns his own successful business, working creatively and constantly and often around the clock. He has a wonderfully dry sense of humor. He is always pleasant, and he seldom gets sick. I admire how he handles his time and energy, and fish. That's right: fish. My friend never carps. He goes fishing. He has been making his own lures lately, which seems like a metaphor for the way he makes his living and his lifestyle. When he can make time, he slips away to an area with mountain streams, taking his big wader boots and his lures.

Then he does very little except enjoy the glory of nature and munch sandwiches. He says there is actually a book about this, by John Gierach, called *Standing in a River, Waving a Stick*.

What are these people doing that works so well to clear their stress and restore them? They are getting away from the rhythmic beat of normal urban life. In a time-out from the constant chafing of the same old stressors of each of their businesses, their pulse rates and cortisol (stress hormone) levels are dropping. They are getting out of the respiratory stress of the city's polluted air. Their energy is going up and their depression is being relieved. They are getting into a cooler climate and into the beauty of nature. They are listening to the sound of rushing water and chattering birds and rustling leaves.

All their senses are now engaged differently than when they are in their typical daily stress situations. They are touching natural surroundings, which raises their DHEA and optimizes their hormonal systems. They are having fun, which makes them laugh and raises endorphin levels. They are experiencing the Divine more directly, being uplifted and refreshed.

Would you trade carping for trout? Is that related to the Latin phrase *carpe diem*? No, silly, that does not mean "carp of the day" or "complaint ritual." It means "seize the day". Until recently, I was always a bit uncomfortable with the *carpe diem* tone in our modern culture. It reminded me of people selfishly grasping: parking places, snacks at a party, someone else's idea. It's almost a sense of "I'd better grab mine now, before the world falls apart".

Personally, I do not believe the world is falling apart at all. I believe we are on the brink of enlightenment and many other good things. I am working hard to be a part of the solutions. Many good people are working hard to be part of the planetary solution set. We are working as well and as fast as we can to put right the matters that must be put right. We are seizing the day in a different way. We are practicing *carpe diem in nomine Domini*, "seize the day in the name of the Lord".

So what are you fishing for in life? Or are you just carping? Figure out what you want to catch, and design your own lures. Then figure out where you need to go and what equipment you need. Keep a delicious sandwich in your pocket. Give yourself some time to stand in a stream waving your stick, letting things develop. Then see what you catch. Throw it back if it isn't what you want, then try other lures. How will you best catch your "fish of the day"? Get going now, and *carpe diem in nomine Domini.*

> **After all, your life is your grand experiment.**
> **What tools will you use?**
> **How far will you go and how high will you rise?**
> **It depends on you.**

# Reflections

# RESOURCES

Britton, Mervin W. 1994. *Willingness: The Driving Force of Accomplishment.* Phoenix: Wentz Publications.

Brown, Nina W. 2001. *Children of the Self-Absorbed.* Oakland, California: New Harbinger Publications.

Callard-Szulgit, *Rosemary. 2003. Perfectionism and Gifted Children.* Lanham, Maryland: Scarecrow Education.

Carter, Jay. 1993. Nasty Men. Columbus: McGraw-Hill.

Carter, Jay. 2003. Nasty People. Columbus: McGraw-Hill Professional.

Forward, Susan with Donna Frazier. 1997. *Emotional Blackmail: When the People in Your Life Use Fear, Obligation, and Guilt to Manipulate You.* NewYork: Quill, An Imprint of Harper-Collins.

Pert, Candace. 1997. *Molecules of Emotion.* New York: Scribner.

Stout, Martha. 2005. *The Sociopath Next Door: The Ruthless and the Rest of Us.* New York: Broadway Books.

## *Discover*
# The Secret Energized You

## Self-Quiz

---

There are 3 ways to use the word "STRESS"

1. as

2. as

3. as

and I now choose #_____! I am now a(n) _____manager!

The most important word to switch is: _____

Instead, I now use:_____


I will now add the following positives to my day:

I will now add the following positives to my week:

Two easy anger-discharge techniques I can use easily are:

1.

2.

My personal morning/evening affirmations are now:

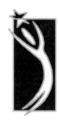

# Kebba Buckley, M.S.
## Healing Therapeutics
(480) 250-1177
*www.kebba.com*
*www.discoverthesecretenergizedyou.com*
2303 N. 44th St. ▲ Suite 14-1181 ▲ Phoenix, AZ 85008-2442

# Order Form

*Date:*_____

*Ship to:*
*Name*_____

*Address*_____

_____

*Phone*_____

*E-mail*_____

| ITEM | PRICE | NUMBER | TOTAL |
|------|-------|--------|-------|
| *Discover The Secret Energized You* | $19.95 each | | |
| | | Subtotal | |
| | | Tax 8.3% | |
| | Shipping @ $3.50 per item | | |
| | | **Total** | |

PAYMENT METHOD:  < > Check  < > Visa  < > MasterCard  < > AmEx

Account
Number_____Expires_____

Signature_____

## *Thank you for your order!*

# About Kebba Buckley

Kebba Buckley is a holistic health educator, pain-solutions therapist, and spiritual teacher who teaches people how to "trade in" their fatigue, stress, and pain for vitality. She sees stress as a sure route to illness, now or later, and energy- and stress management through personal balance as the primary key to wellness. Kebba is known as The LifeTools Lady. She gives people tools for feeling energized and wonderful instead of tired, tight, or in direct physical pain.

Kebba works with groups and with individuals, teaching practical, memorable techniques for satisfied living: physical movements, breath techniques, emotional methods, mental processes, and spiritual approaches. She emphasizes oriental and yogic philosophy and energy balancing in addition to standard Western models and modalities. Kebba's background includes Sensitivity Training and Omega Vector Training. She sees personal responsibility and choice of state as vital components of personal energy management.

Kebba has both A.B. and M.S. degrees in sciences. She spent sixteen years in both government and consulting engineering. A workaholic manager during those years, she discovered a number of health issues that medical doctors had no answers for. She thus became an energetic researcher of methods for managing the stress/energy balance and its impact on health. A certified instructor of Jin Shin Jyutsu for self-help, Kebba has had a Jin Shin Jyutsu practice and has offered personal-growth seminars since 1985. She was ordained in 2000 and teaches meditation and spiritual-growth seminars.

Kebba's columns, *UpBeat Living* and *StressTips!*, have appeared in *One Planet* magazine, *ec Magazine*, and *Much Ado About Mensa*. She is the creator of the Half-Minute Stress Management Method$^{sm}$, the UpBeat Living Energy Equation$^{sm}$, and the RELF YourSelf$^{sm}$ technique. She has given seminars for such diverse groups as the American Association of Public Welfare Attorneys, American Mensa Ltd., American Business Women's' Association (ABWA), Business Networks International (BNI), Desert Christian Fellowship (Phoenix, AZ), IMPACT for Enterprising Women (Phoenix, AZ), Palo Cristi Presbyterian Church (Paradise Valley, AZ), Unity Business Network (Phoenix, AZ), Unity of Phoenix, and the law firm of Brobeck, Pfleger, and Harrison (San Francisco, CA).

# Reflections